# Shining Light on Constipation

## Rectal Descent and Other Colon, Rectal and Anal Problems

**FIRST EDITION**

By Christopher J. Lahr, M. D., F. A. C. S.
Complete Colon Care PC
Carolina Constipation Center
2097 Henry Tecklenburg Drive, Suite 311
Charleston SC 29414
Tel: 843-763-3592 • Fax: 843-763-4171

*with contributions by*

Elizabeth T. Clerico, R.N., M.S.
Bon Secours St. Francis Xavier Hospital
Charleston SC 29414

# Acknowledgments

I would like to thank my wife, Debbie Frei-Lahr, MD, for putting up with my long hours at the hospital and office on weekdays, and my long hours at a computer on the weekends, and for taking care of Kelley and Derek while I am away. I thank Barbara Shaw, CMA, who orchestrates my office and encourages me to use my computer skills, and Vicki Limehouse who assists me with all my patients. Mona Small, Barbara Bates and Carlene Hanckel keep my office running smoothly and enable me to see as many patients as I do. Beth Clerico, RN, performs and reads all of my pelvic floor physiology studies and assists patients with pelvic muscle retraining.

Christopher J. Lahr
February 1997

**Shining Light on Constipation: Rectal Descent and Other Colon, Rectal and Anal Problems**

Copyright © Dr. Christopher J. Lahr

First Edition – April 1997
Fourth Printing – November 1998

**ISBN 0-9648176-3-2**

Published by TRIAD Services, Inc., Charleston, South Carolina U.S.A.

While every precaution has been taken in the preparation of this book, the author and publisher assume no responsibility or liability for errors or omissions, or for any damages resulting from the use of the contents of this book.

# Shining Light on Constipation
## Rectal Descent and Other Colon, Rectal and Anal Problems

### TABLES OF CONTENTS

# LIST OF FIGURES

# A Personal Note from the Author

People often ask how I got started in the colon business. Born into a military family, through the U.S. Air Force I attended medical school at the University of Alabama in Birmingham. In my fifth and final year, I realized that as a general surgeon without any specialty skills, the Air Force would probably send me to a small hospital. If I wanted to go to a bigger hospital or medical center I would have to have a specialty.

One day I got an Air Force brochure in the mail that said the Air Force needed surgeons specializing in cardiothoracic, pediatric, vascular, and colorectal surgery. I chose colorectal surgery. The University of Minnesota in St. Paul, Minnesota accepted me into its colon and rectal surgery fellowship.

How I became interested in constipation is a little more complicated, but it started in Minnesota. While I was a colon and rectal surgery fellow, we saw many patients with anal sphincter problems such as leakage. I decided it would be useful to be able to take an X-ray picture of the anal sphincter muscles while measuring their strength.

I developed a sphincterography balloon to do this. I made the first ones out of rubber drains, Sears garden hose connectors, and silk thread. Tubing connected the balloon to a bag of X-ray dye. The higher the bag, the higher the pressure in the balloon. We watched the balloon in the patient with X-rays. We could see how strong the sphincter was by seeing how much X-ray dye it could squeeze out of the balloon at different pressures.

I modified the balloon to show people their sphincter pressure. We could train them to squeeze and to relax. They could strengthen their muscle against the balloon. I patented these balloons, hoping they would make me a millionaire. After I had a patent, I formed Sunburst Biomedical Corporation with a partner. For the next four years, I traveled around the country in my spare time selling Lahr Balloons.

Eventually I came to two harsh realities: I was never going to get rich selling Lahr Balloons; and there was not widespread interest in constipation and incontinence.

By the time I learned these lessons, I had full-time private practice in Charleston, South Carolina. I was so confident of the importance of treating constipation and incontinence, that I limited my practice to these problems. I didn't treat colon cancer, diverticulitis, or other colon problems unrelated to constipation.

A two year reality bath left me with substantial debts and the realization that I could not cure all constipation and incontinence with biofeedback and the Lahr Balloon. I was disappointed with how things had turned out. Not only was I having difficulty treating constipation successfully, I did not get many patients referred for anything else.

For two years I treated many anal problems, hemorrhoids, fissures, anal pain, rectal pain, and rectal bleeding and did a lot of colonoscopies for rectal bleeding, constipation and abdominal pain. I saw many patients that other doctors had been unable to help. Often they were referred to me just before or after they were sent to a psychiatrist. These patients had various combinations of abdominal pain and constipation. They all had normal colonoscopies. I studied them all with the Lahr Balloon, intestinal transit time measurement and defecography, but could not help very many. I was able to help some of the patients with very slow colons by shortening the colon.

This is where things stood in 1994. It took several steps to come to a better understanding of surgery for constipation. With each step, there was a patient that taught me something new.

In 1994, a local colon surgeon sent "Betty" to me with rectal bleeding, rectal pain, lower abdominal pain and difficult rectal emptying. Betty didn't have just a little rectal bleeding. Before I met her she had bled into shock and had a near-death experience. She had been admitted to intensive care and had been given seven units of blood transfusions for the bleeding. All they could find were some bleeding hemorrhoids. They sewed these up. Shortly thereafter, she saw me for the first time.

She continued to bleed, and the front of the lower part of her rectum was always raw. I thought it might be Crohn's disease (colonic inflammation) but the biopsies never confirmed it. Her defecography (X-ray of the rectum during emptying) showed a long flat rectum lying low in the pelvis with a forward bulge (rectocele) into the vagina.

Finally, in the operating room, I took some deep biopsies of the raw area. The pathologist looked at these and said she had a solitary rectal ulcer. A solitary rectal ulcer is a pressure sore in the front of the rectum that happens when the front of the rectum is pushed down into the anal canal. This blocks the opening, and makes it very difficult to empty the rectum. The treatment is a little controversial, but I had treated two solitary rectal ulcers in the past by shortening the colon just above the rectum (sigmoidectomy), and lifting the rectum up and sewing it to the lower backbone (rectopexy).

By this time Betty said she would rather have a colostomy bag then go on living with the rectal pain and difficult rectal emptying she was having. I decided it was worth a try. I did the sigmoidectomy and rectopexy, and she got better. She was able to move her bowels without straining, her pain resolved, and she stopped bleeding.

A month later I saw another woman with similar complaints. She could not empty her rectum. She had bad rectal pain and constipation, but she did not have rectal bleeding. When I examined her rectum, she did not have a solitary rectal ulcer. However, the moment I saw her defecography a light went on in my head. Her defecography looked just like Betty's. It was flat and low, and bulged over the vagina. The lower end of the rectum snapped shut before the upper rectum was empty. Her colon was slow, so we planned an operation to shorten it. While doing that surgery, I lifted up the rectum and sewed it to the sacrum (lower backbone). Though she wasn't perfect after surgery, she was better and I had crossed a mental bridge. I had seen a rectal shape on defecography that looked just like the rectal shape of patients with solitary rectal ulcers. This patient didn't have the ulcer, but she did have the difficult rectal emptying. Her rectal emptying improved when I did a solitary rectal ulcer operation (sigmoidectomy and rectopexy).

I realized that I had been seeing this rectal shape for years in patients with difficult rectal emptying, but I had not known what it meant or what to do about it. I now thought that their difficult rectal emptying was due to the rectum sliding down into the pelvis, probably during pregnancy and childbirth. Since lifting the rectum up and shortening the sigmoid colon relieved the symptoms, it must be the extra length and the rectal descent into the pelvis which caused the difficult rectal emptying. If so, then by identifying the women with this particular rectal shape and doing a sigmoidectomy and rectopexy, I could correct their rectal emptying difficulties.

I have now done 50 operations for rectal descent. I have written about it and sent abstracts (reports) to medical societies. I have done over 50 operations to shorten the colon to treat severe constipation. I have added to the rectopexy operation. Now I also lift up the vagina and support it from the sacrum. This supports the front of the rectum as well.

We have interviewed all the people who have had this rectal descent surgery. Here are their answers to some of our questions.

*Shining Light on Constipation*

1. How satisfied are you with the surgery?
   | | | |
   |---|---|---|
   | Extremely | 31 | (67%) |
   | Very | 9 | (20%) |
   | Satisfied | 3 | (7%) |
   | Neutral | 2 | (4%) |
   | Not satisfied | 1 | (2%) |

2. How often do you strain?
   | | | |
   |---|---|---|
   | Never | 15 | (33%) |
   | Rarely | 9 | (20%) |
   | Occasionally | 11 | (24%) |
   | Often | 7 | (15%) |
   | Usually | 4 | (9%) |

3. How Hard is the Straining?
   | | | |
   |---|---|---|
   | None | 14 | (30%) |
   | Slight | 12 | (26%) |
   | Moderate | 11 | (24%) |
   | Hard | 1 | (2%) |
   | Very Hard | 8 | (17%) |

4. How much easier are bowel movements now?
   | | | |
   |---|---|---|
   | Markedly Better | 35 | (76%) |
   | Improved | 4 | (9%) |
   | Slightly easier | 5 | 11%) |
   | Not Improved | 1 | (2%) |
   | Worse | 1 | (2%) |

Though it is not perfect we are definitely improving rectal emptying with surgery. We continue to try to improve our results and our surgical techniques. My goal is to perfect the surgery for constipation for those individuals who do not respond to other measures.

# 1

# What You Can do to Help Yourself

Hard bowel movements and loose bowel movements cause many colon and rectal problems. Small hard bowel movements cut and tear the anal lining. They drag the rectal lining out. Loose or semi-liquid bowel movements do not open the anal canal properly. They stick to and irritate the anal skin. Bowel movements should not be too hard, too soft, or too small. If bowel movements are the right size and consistency, many colon rectal complaints will disappear.

There are two simple things you can do to clear up many anal and colon problems. These two simple health measures are: 1) taking natural vegetable powder daily, and 2) practicing water hygiene.

The simplest, and usually the only way to give bowel movements the proper consistency, is by eating fiber. Fiber acts as a stool normalizer. It prevents the stools from being too hard or too soft. It helps the bowels move one to three times a day, which is good for the anus. It prevents stools from tearing the anal skin and will prevent bowel movements from dragging the rectal lining out of the rectum. Fiber helps the bowel movements slip out more easily by making the feces less sticky. This helps to prevent them from adhering to the anal skin.

## Natural Vegetable Powder

Drugstores sell natural vegetable powder (psyllium) without a prescription. Natural vegetable powder comes in sugar-free and low-grit varieties; both are fine to use. It is sold under many names and brands including Natural Fiber Laxative, Metamucil, and Natural Vegetable Powder. Citrucel is also a fiber supplement, though it does not contain psyllium.

---

However, Citrucel does not cause as much gas and bloating in some people, and it can be used by persons allergic to psyllium.

The recommended dose on the back of the bottle often does not clear up most anal problems. Therefore, I recommend a dose of *three heaping tablespoonfuls* (not teaspoonfuls) in water, juice or milk once each morning. Drink it as soon as you stir it, otherwise it will turn into a thick porridge.

Some special "smooth" brands of psyllium add sugar and may not contain as much psyllium fiber per tablespoon. Therefore, you may have to take more. Read the label on the bottle to determine how many tablespoons are needed to equal at least 10 grams. This is needed as a supplement to your diet. Because one's total daily fiber intake should be 25-35 grams, a high-fiber diet (in addition to the supplement) will ensure that you get as much fiber as you need.

Some people experience cramps when they first start using natural vegetable powder. If this should happen, cut the dose in half for one week, and then return to the regular dose of three heaping tablespoonfuls each morning.

When taking psyllium be sure to drink additional fluids whenever you are thirsty. Six to eight full glasses of water or juice daily is recommended.

Even if you think your bowels move all right, take the natural vegetable powder anyway. Try it and see. You will notice a difference in less than a week.

## Water Hygiene

Most Americans use dry toilet paper to wipe the anal area after moving their bowels. This smears the feces (bowel movement material) over the anal skin. The more a person wipes, the more the feces is rubbed into the skin. This causes itching and irritation. To prevent these problems, use water hygiene after each bowel movement.

Water hygiene can be accomplished in several different ways. One way is to use a small squirt bottle like a mustard or catsup bottle used in restaurants. (Be sure you have your own clean bottle. You do not literally want to use the catsup bottle.) Fill the bottle with clean warm water, and squirt the water onto the anal area. You can also use a bulb syringe to do the same thing. Then, use dry toilet paper to blot the skin dry without wiping. If there is any brown material on the toilet paper, wash again with water and continue to do so until the blotting paper stays clean.

Another option is to use a warm, wet cloth to cleanse yourself after each bowel movement. Then, gently blot the skin with paper to dry and check for any additional soiling.

If you keep your toilet bowl very clean and do not put any chemicals into the water, you may use water from the toilet bowl for water hygiene. To do this, flush the toilet after your bowel movement. Do not wipe yourself. Instead, lift up the toilet seat, lean over the toilet and use your hand to splash the clean water onto the anal area. Use dry toilet paper to gently blot the area dry. If there is any soiling still on the paper, splash with water and dry again until the paper is clean.

Make a plan for how you will accomplish water hygiene in a public restroom. You may want to keep a small wet cloth in a ziplock plastic bag. Or, if you prefer, you can buy commercially packaged wet "wipes" (cloths) to keep in your purse or pocket. If you do this, look for labels that say "no alcohol, hypoallergenic, fragrance free."

## Conclusions

Natural vegetable powder and a large amount of fiber in the diet help to make a bowel movement that is easy to pass and causes a minimal amount of soiling. Be sure to also use some method of water hygiene after each bowel movement to assure that the anal area stays clean. This will reduce any potential for irritation, itching, or other problems.

# What are the Colon, Rectum and Anus?

The intestines are long, hollow tubes that run from your stomach to your anal opening. There are two intestines: the small and the large. This size designation refers to circumference; the "small" intestine is about 25 feet long. It is about as big around as your middle finger. It absorbs the nutrition from your food. The small intestine empties into the large intestine, also called the colon, which is about 5 or 6 feet long. The colon is about an inch or two in diameter and connects your small intestine to your anus. The large intestine absorbs water and stores the waste-products of digestion until your body is ready to empty them out.

The large intestine is shaped like a large question mark and starts out near your right hip, moves up to your ribs on the right side, goes across to the left side by your ribs, then down to the left hip where it makes an S-curve down to the anus. The last portion of the colon is called the rectum. At the bottom of the rectum are the sphincter muscles. There are internal and external anal sphincter muscles. These muscles prevent the rectum from emptying when you do not want it to.

Problems of the colon, rectum and anus include colon cancer, hemorrhoids, colon polyps, constipation, diverticulitis, colitis, Crohn's disease, diarrhea, incontinence (leakage), rectal pain, and difficult rectal emptying. We will discuss all of these starting with anal problems.

## Anal Problems

Most anal and rectal problems are *not* due to colon cancers. Rectal bleeding, pain, itching, and swelling or lumps in the anal area are often due to hemorrhoids or other benign problems of the anal area.

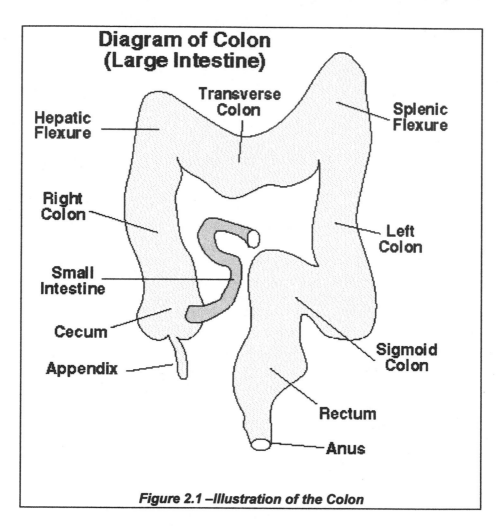

**Diagram of Colon
(Large Intestine)**

Figure 2.1 –Illustration of the Colon

The anal canal is one to two inches long. It is surrounded by the anal sphincter muscles which squeeze the anal canal closed to make sure that stool does not leak out accidentally. When a person is ready to move his bowels, he relaxes these sphincter muscles and strains down to push the stool out.

The rectum and the upper half of the anal canal are lined with mucosa, a thin velvety layer of tissue similar to that which lines the rest of the intestines. The lower one-half of the anal canal is lined with skin. This skin is very sensitive to pain. The anal mucosa is not sensitive to pain, but it is sensitive to being stretched or tugged.

There are small crypts or little glands in the lining of the anal canal which secrete oil. Stool has a tendency to get caught in the crypts if the stool (feces) is hard and if a person has to strain hard to move his bowels. The high pressure from straining forces the stool into the crypts. If feces gets trapped in these little crypts, it can fester there and cause infections, abscesses and fistulas.

Some common problems in this area include pruritus (itching), fissures (cracks in the anal skin), external hemorrhoids (blood blisters under the anal skin), internal hemorrhoids (when the rectal lining gets dragged out of the rectum), fistulas (tunnels from the rectum or anal canal to the skin that can drain pus), and abscesses (pus pockets).

## Anal Itching

*Pruritus ani* (anal itching) is a rash or irritation of the anal skin. The skin just outside the anal opening is raw and chapped. There may be little ulcers or sores on the anal skin. This can cause severe itching, burning and even pain.

*Pruritus* is not due to an infection. It is not due to a cancer, and it will not turn into cancer. It is caused by the irritation of the anal skin by chemicals in the stool and in soaps.

When toilet paper is used to wipe the anal area after bowel movements, it has a tendency to smear some of the bowel movement material over the anal skin. Dry toilet paper cannot remove all of this stool material. Therefore, it leaves a thin layer on the anal skin which dries and irritates the skin. This dryness and irritation of the anal skin can be made *worse* by soaps and vigorous washing.

Pruritus ani can be very painful and uncomfortable and can last a long time. Fortunately, it is fairly easy to treat with the use of natural vegetable powder taken daily in liquid, and with the practice of water hygiene. In addition, Vaseline or petroleum jelly can be applied to the anal region 1, 2 or 3 times a day to decrease the symptoms.

Soap aggravates itching. One of the most important things in reducing the pruritus is to stop using soaps to wash the anal area. Soap removes the natural oils from the anal skin and this makes the dryness worse. However, if you feel you must use soap, try to use it less often, and use a moisturizing skin care bar (such as Tone or Dove) which is less likely to remove the natural oils of the skin.

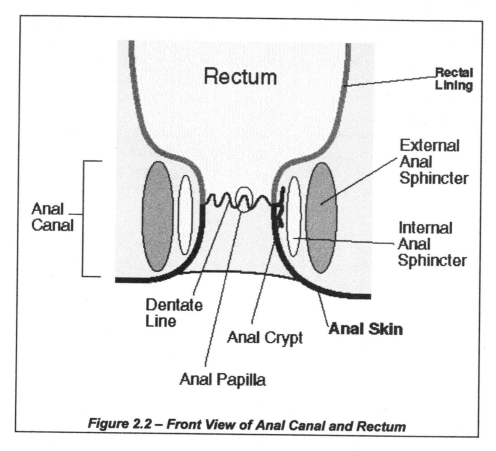

**Figure 2.2 – Front View of Anal Canal and Rectum**

## Fissures

Fissures are cracks in the anal skin caused by small or hard bowel movements.   Diarrhea can also cause fissures by drying out the skin until it cracks open (just as dish water can cause cracks in the skin of the hands). Since anal skin is very sensitive, these cracks can cause severe pain.  They can also cause anal bleeding. The pain and bleeding is worse after bowel movements. Usually, the bleeding is bright red.

Occasionally, fissures are very large, ugly and raw. In this case, they may be due to Crohn's disease, an inflammation of the lining of the colon. Crohn's disease will be discussed later in this book.

Natural vegetable powder will cure at least half of all fissures.  If the pain is extremely bad, or if the fissures do not disappear as a result of fiber therapy, they can be cured by simple outpatient surgery.

In this surgery, a small quarter inch to one-half inch incision is made in the anal skin near the anal fissure. The incision is made over the internal anal sphincter muscle. Once the incision is made in the skin, some of the muscle fibers of the internal sphincter are divided. This releases the tension off of the skin at the anal fissure. This allows the fissure to heal as the skin closes. If swollen skin and scar tissue are present at the fissure, these may also be removed. Individuals can usually be back to work 2 to 10 days after their surgery.

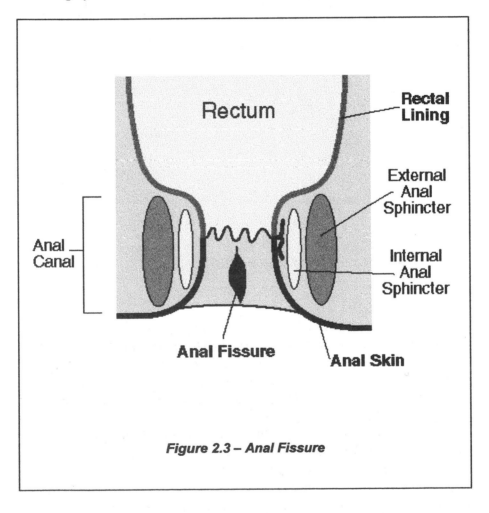

*Figure 2.3 – Anal Fissure*

# 3

# Hemorrhoids, Fistulas and Abscesses

## External Thrombosed Hemorrhoids

Thrombosed external hemorrhoids are blood blisters under the skin of the anal opening. Bowel movements that are too hard scrape across the anal skin and cause a shearing action. This causes the blood vessels below the skin to tear. The stronger skin above is left intact.

The blood vessel which has been torn open leaks blood under the skin and forms a blood clot (thrombosis). This is not dangerous to the rest of the body. However, because it stretches the skin and the nerve endings in the anal skin, it causes severe pain and swelling.

Usually, a thrombosed external hemorrhoid does not cause bleeding unless the skin over the blood clot gets rubbed away. Then, the blood clot can ooze out and cause bleeding.

Thrombosed external hemorrhoids will resolve in four-to-six weeks as the blood clot is re-absorbed by the body. They are generally most tender in the first four days. If the thrombosis is quite painful and has been present for less than 4 days, then surgical excision (removal) is the best treatment. If the thrombosis has been present for more than four days, and is beginning to resolve, it is generally better to leave it alone.

The choice of treatment also depends upon how severe the pain is. If the pain is quite severe and the person finds it difficult to walk, work or sleep, then excising (removing) the clot and the blood vessel will result in quicker relief and improvement. If the pain is relatively mild, the pain seems to be getting better, and the thrombosis seems to be shrinking, then it is best to leave the thrombosis alone and let it resolve by itself.

Removing the hemorrhoid is a fairly simple procedure. The area of the hemorrhoid is cleaned with a betadine or alcohol solution. Marcaine, which is an anesthetic agent like Novocain, is injected around the thrombosed hemorrhoid. The thrombosis (blood clot), the blood vessel, and the skin over the blood clot, are then removed. Generally, no stitches are required. A gauze dressing is applied. Pain pills may be needed for the first few days. The pain from thrombosed hemorrhoids and fissures is generally much improved immediately after surgery.

## Internal Hemorrhoids

The mucosal lining of the anal canal and rectum is soft and fragile, velvet-like in its appearance and texture. It is very sensitive to being stretched. Passing hard or small bowel movements causes the anal and rectal mucosa to become stretched. If the stretched mucosa is dragged outside of the anal canal, it forms what is called an internal hemorrhoid. Internal hemorrhoids may be painful, and they may bleed.

Internal hemorrhoids can be pushed back up inside the anal canal. This reduces the pain and slows down the bleeding. If a person must use his hand to push hemorrhoids back up inside after each bowel movement, he has internal, not external, hemorrhoids.

## Treatments for Internal Hemorrhoids

Treatments for internal hemorrhoids include natural vegetable powder, infrared coagulation, rubber band ligation, laser excision and surgical excision.

*Natural vegetable powder* will create soft, formed, and good-sized bowel movements which will stretch the anal opening to its proper size so that the mucosa will not be dragged out of the anal canal. This can result in improvement or complete disappearance of the internal hemorrhoids If natural vegetable powder alone does not help, and bleeding and protrusion continues, then the excess mucosa which has been dragged out must be removed surgically. This can be done using any one of several techniques.

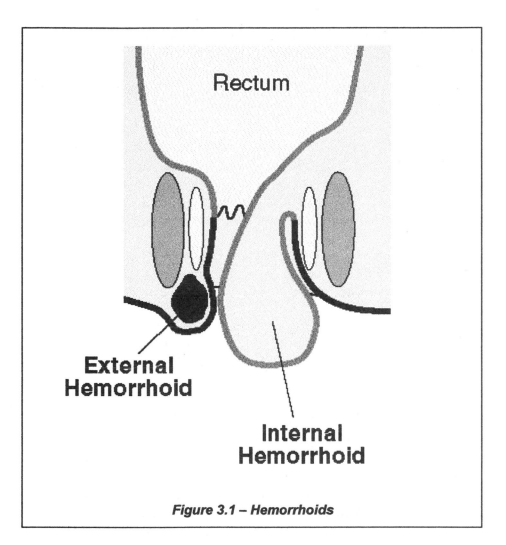

**Figure 3.1 – Hemorrhoids**

*Infrared Coagulation* is the simplest technique. An infrared light beam burns away some of the excess mucosal lining. This procedure can be done in the doctor's office. It does not require anesthesia. It does not cause any significant pain. Remember, the anal mucosa is sensitive only to being stretched. This treatment works best when there are only small areas of excess hemorrhoidal mucosa to be removed.

*Rubber Band Ligation* is done if somewhat larger amounts of internal hemorrhoidal mucosa must be removed. A special instrument will place a small rubber band around a lump of mucosa about the size of a raisin or small grape. The rubber band cuts off the blood supply (circulation), and within four to 10 days, the hemorrhoid falls off. Sometimes, when the hemorrhoid falls off, there is some bleeding. It is generally not severe. If a person is on blood thinners such as Coumadin, rubber band ligation is not used because of the potential for bleeding.

In a small number of cases (about 1 in 5,000), serious infection develops in the anal area which requires a further treatment with antibiotics and, occasionally, surgery. If a person has the rubber band treatment and develops a fever, severe pain or difficulty urinating, the person should see a doctor immediately. In most cases, rubber band ligation is simple and painless, and can be done in the doctor's office without the need to miss work.

NOTE: Rubber bands cannot be used to treat external hemorrhoids since the anal skin is very sensitive to pain.

## Surgery for Hemorrhoids

Some internal hemorrhoids protrude so far and become so large, that they cannot be removed with either rubber band ligation or infrared coagulation. This is especially true if the internal hemorrhoids are also associated with swollen or protruding skin. Surgery may be indicated since the skin cannot be removed with rubber bands. In addition, only a limited number of internal hemorrhoids can be removed with rubber bands one at a time. So, surgery may be indicated.

The important factor to consider is how much trouble the hemorrhoids are causing. If the hemorrhoids are not causing very much trouble in the way of pain or bleeding, and if the person does not mind waiting several months for treatment to be completed, then rubber band ligation or infrared coagulation are considered.

If the internal hemorrhoids are causing a great deal of pain, discomfort, protrusion, and bleeding, or the person does not wish to wait several months for treatment to be completed, then surgery is indicated. The advantage of surgery is that all of the hemorrhoids can be treated at one time. The disadvantage is that while some people have been able to return to work after one week, others will require two to three weeks of recuperation before they feel able to return to work.

This surgery can be completed using local anesthesia, spinal block, or general anesthesia. When local anesthesia is used, the surgeon gives medications by vein so that the patient sleeps through the procedure and does not feel or remember any of the procedure. This is the safest type of anesthesia.

After he gives the anesthesia, the surgeon places a metal scope into the anal canal to see the internal hemorrhoids. He lifts up the excess hemorrhoidal mucosa and removes the bulging internal and external hemorrhoids with scissors or a laser beam. The laser is more expensive than the scissors. There is no difference in the amount of pain afterwards or the outcome of the surgery.

After removing the internal and external hemorrhoids, the surgeon sews the anal and rectal mucosa to the underlying muscle so that it cannot protrude again. He carefully avoids injury to any of the sphincter muscles underneath the hemorrhoids.

The suture (surgical thread) will dissolve, and does not have to be removed later. This is outpatient surgery. The person has the surgery in the afternoon and goes home the next morning.

After hemorrhoid surgery, it is important to take three heaping tablespoons of natural vegetable powder daily so the bowels move easily with less pain. Warm baths help reduce the pain following surgery as do Sitz baths, which spray water on the anal area.

It is normal to have some bleeding after hemorrhoid surgery, but if it is more than one half cup, the patient should call the surgeon.

## Fistulas and Abscesses

We have already described the small crypts, or little glands, in the lining of the anal canal which secrete oil. Stool has a tendency to get caught in the crypts if the stool (feces) is hard, and if a person has to strain hard to move his bowels. The high pressure from straining forces the stool into the crypts. Feces trapped in these little crypts can fester and cause infections, abscesses and fistulas.

Abscesses are pockets of pus within the flesh, which can cause fistulas. Fistulas are tunnels through the flesh from the anal canal to the skin. Fistulas can cause chronic discharge or drainage. The abscesses are extremely painful, swollen and tender.

Abscesses should be treated as soon as possible so that they do not damage the anal sphincter muscles. Antibiotics alone usually do not help, because antibiotics cannot get into the abscess cavity which is filled with pus. Surgery is required to drain abscesses. An abscess close to the skin can be drained in the doctor's office. For a deep abscess, surgery must be done in the hospital.

Fistulas must be opened up with surgery. How big the surgical opening must be is determined by how deep and complicated the fistula is.

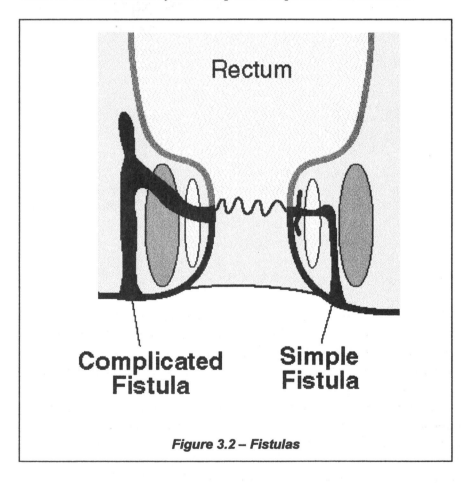

**Figure 3.2 – Fistulas**

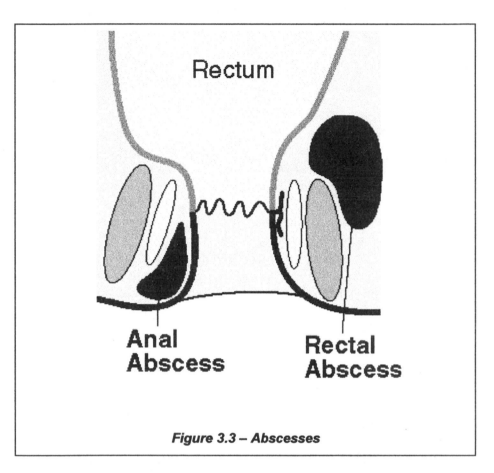

**Figure 3.3 – Abscesses**

Sometimes a fistula involves the anus or a large amount of sphincter muscle. When this occurs, rather than cut the muscle to open the fistula up, the surgeon simply passes a rubberband, called a seton, through the fistula and leaves it loosely tied in place. This allows the pus to drain so that the fistula can heal.

Sometimes, additional surgery must be done after the fistula has healed, to close up the inside hole of the fistula. If needed, a flap of rectal mucosa and internal anal sphincter muscle can be used to close the internal opening of the fistula after the seton is removed. The setons are usually temporary, although sometimes the surgeon may leave them in for as long as six to twelve months. For simple fistulas, setons are usually left in place only a few weeks or months.

## Rectovaginal Fistulas

A rectovaginal fistula is a tunnel which develops between the rectum and vagina. It may be caused by an injury during the vaginal delivery of babies or by an infection. When this happens, gas from the bowel or stool from the rectum can enter the vagina through the tunnel. This results in infections in the vaginal area. It can also cause poor control over the passage of gas or stool from the rectum. The only way to close the fistula is with surgery.

This can be done in one of two ways. One method opens the fistula up. The surgeon frees up the sphincter muscles and re-wraps them around the anal opening. He wraps the sphincter muscle across the fistula which closes the defect. The skin is left open to prevent infection. The wound closes up completely in four to eight weeks.

Another method pulls a flap of the rectal mucosa and internal anal sphincter down over the fistula opening. This requires a three to seven day hospital stay. The person is usually sore for two to six weeks following the surgery.

## Impactions

Impactions are hard lumps of stool that get caught in the rectum. The person feels as if there is something that is falling down onto the anal canal and blocking it. There may also be pain or feelings of pressure in the pelvic area. A person with an impaction can treat himself at home by using enemas. Impactions that are not removed through the use of enemas can usually be broken up in the physician's office. Once the impaction is broken up it can be washed out using enemas. The long term treatment for impactions is natural vegetable powder.

The simplest and safest enema to use can be made at home with a simple recipe. Mix one pint of lukewarm water with 1 tablespoon of sugar and one teaspoon of salt. This solution is inserted into the rectum using an enema tip with an enema bag or an enema bottle.

## Rectal Bleeding

Rectal bleeding is a very common symptom or complaint that can be divided into two categories. There is outside (external) bleeding and there is inside (internal) bleeding.

External bleeding comes from outside of the rectum, from the anal skin or anal canal. It looks bright red on the toilet paper; or, if it drips into the toilet bowl, it is always bright red. There is no blood mixed in with the bowel movements. The person has no bloody diarrhea and does not pass any blood clots.

Internal rectal bleeding comes from the rectum or colon, or even from the small intestine or the stomach. This bleeding is associated with blood clots, blood mixed in with bowel movements, dark purple blood, black stools, bloody diarrhea, or bleeding associated with belly pain. Sometimes, the blood is hidden and can only be seen by doing a special hemoccult test. If internal rectal bleeding occurs, the person should be evaluated with a colonoscopy to determine the cause of the bleeding.

Sometimes it is impossible to tell if the rectal bleeding is internal or external and further testing such as colonoscopy must be done. (Colonoscopy is described later in this book).

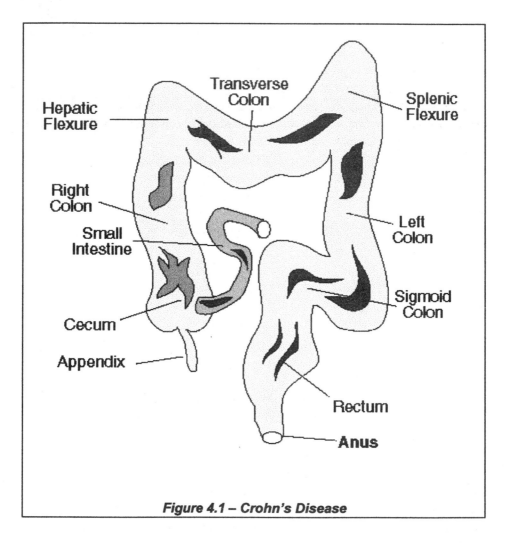

*Figure 4.1 – Crohn's Disease*

# Colitis and Crohn's Disease

J ust as some people get arthritis which is an inflammation of the joints, it
is also possible to get inflammation of the colon. Inflammation of the
colon (large intestine) is called colitis. Germs can cause colitis. Poor
blood supply can cause colitis. Some medications can cause colitis.
However, in **most** cases, the cause of colitis is not known.

When no other cause can be found for the inflammation, it falls into one
of two categories: ulcerative colitis or Crohn's colitis (Crohn's disease of the
colon). Diet and psychological factors do not cause ulcerative colitis or
Crohn's disease. No germs have been found to cause these conditions.
Colitis is not infectious; it cannot be passed from one person to another like
the flu or a common cold.

## Ulcerative Colitis versus Crohn's Disease

Ulcerative colitis causes inflammation only in the mucosal (superficial)
lining of the colon. It does not affect the small intestine or the stomach.
Ulcerative colitis generally starts in the rectum and spreads from the rectum
toward the first part of the colon in a steady progression.

Crohn's disease involves the entire thickness of the wall of the colon, and
can also involve other parts of the intestines such as the small intestine.
Since Crohn's disease can involve the entire thickness of the intestine,
sometimes long ulcers are seen in the colon lining. These ulcers look as if
someone had pulled a grass rake across the lining of the colon. They are
called rake ulcers or bear claw ulcers. Crohn's disease can be patchy. It can
be present in one part of the colon, absent in another, and then present in the
next part.

Crohn's disease involves the small intestine, but ulcerative colitis does
not. The last one to two feet of the small intestine are called the ileum. If

---

ulcers and extensive inflammation are seen in the ileum the colitis may be due to Crohn's disease.

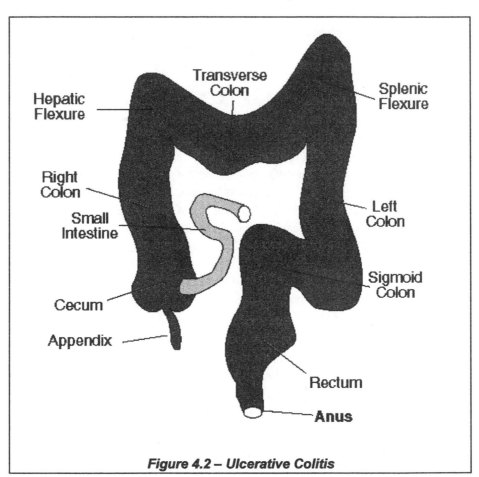

**Figure 4.2 – Ulcerative Colitis**

The colitis associated with Crohn's disease is often associated with anal problems such as fissures, fistulas, abscesses and skin tags; whereas, ulcerative colitis never causes anal problems.

When Crohn's disease involves the small intestine it can cause narrowing of the small intestine, called strictures. It can also cause a complete blockage. Ulcerative colitis never involves the small intestine.

Ulcerative colitis can be cured by removing the entire colon if necessary. Crohn's disease can never be completely cured. If areas of the small intestine or colon which are involved with the Crohn's disease are removed, the surgery will generally relieve the person's symptoms for a while, sometimes for many years. However, at some point in the future, symptoms may recur.

Whether colitis is due to ulcerative colitis or Crohn's disease is generally not important unless surgery is required. If surgery is required, then ulcerative colitis is treated differently than Crohn's colitis. If surgery is not required, ulcerative colitis is generally treated with medications in the same manner as is Crohn's colitis.

## Medicines for Colitis

The treatments for colitis due to ulcerative colitis or Crohn's colitis include many medications which decrease inflammation. These include: Prednisone, other steroids, Imuran (azathioprine) and Cyclosporin. There are also a number of other medications which relieve the colitis, including Azulfidine, Dipentum, Asacol, Rowasa suppositories and Rowasa enemas.

Azulfidine (sulfasalazine) was one of the early medications used against colitis, and is still quite effective. Azulfidine is a pill. It has been used many years and is less expensive than some of the newer pills. It does have some side effects which are not present in the newer medications. For example, it may cause low blood counts, headaches, kidney problems, and a serious skin rash. It cannot be taken by people with a sulfa allergy.

New medications such as Dipentum, Asacol and Pentasa have the same active ingredients as Azulfidine, but they do not cause problems in people with sulfa allergies. These pills are taken by mouth, and reduce inflammation in the intestine.

If the inflammation is only in the rectum, then Rowasa suppositories can be used. These suppositories contain the same active ingredient found in Azulfidine, Pentasa, Asacol and Dipentum. However, because Rowasa is a suppository, the medication is applied directly to the inflamed area of the rectum.

If the inflammation involves only the bottom two feet, that is, the left side of the colon and the rectum, then Rowasa enemas can be used. These enemas also contain the same active ingredient as Azulfidine, Asacol and Dipentum, but apply it directly to the lining of the colon.

The pills and the enemas or suppositories can be used together. Often suppositories or enemas are used to get the colitis under control. Then, they are gradually tapered off, and the person continues to take one of the pills.

The next line of therapy involves the use of steroids. Prednisone is the main steroid used in the treatment of colitis. Prednisone is fairly inexpensive. When taken in high doses, it has side effects which include lessened immunity to infections, weight gain, nervousness and mental hyperactivity, some emotional changes, facial changes or fattening, and stretch marks on the skin. These side effects generally occur only if the steroids are used for more than a few weeks. Usually, the steroids are used in high doses for only a few days or weeks, to gain control of the disease. Then, their use is tapered off over a week or two. The colitis is then controlled by using a pill such as Dipentum or Asacol, with or without the enemas or suppositories. Sometimes steroids must be used longer.

If the medications do not control the colitis or if the side effects from the medical treatment become intolerable, then physicians consider surgery. Symptoms of colitis include rectal bleeding, abdominal pain, diarrhea, passage of mucus and bloody stools. Indications for surgery include rupture of the colon, severe bleeding, very frequent diarrhea, severe weight loss and chronic illness which never gets better.

## Ileal Pouch for Ulcerative Colitis

A new surgical technique, developed within the last 20 years, can cure ulcerative colitis without the need for a colostomy or ileostomy bag. The Ileal Pouch technique is a surgical procedure which removes the entire colon, from the point of its attachment at the small intestine to the point of its attachment at the anus. The anal sphincter muscles and the anus are left intact. The last 10 inches of the small intestine (the ileum) are then used to make a U-shaped sac (pouch) which is attached to the anus at the anal opening.

This pouch acts as a new rectum. The anal sphincter is left in place so that the person can still control his bowel movements. A person generally moves his bowels 4 to 8 times per day following this operation. However, he has reasonably good control, and no longer has any symptoms of the colitis.

The ileal pouch procedure requires two operations. During the first operation, the surgeon removes the entire colon, creates the pouch and hooks it to the anus. He makes an ileostomy, which means that the person must temporarily wear a bag on the abdomen to collect stool. This prevents bowel contents from entering the pouch until it is healed. After about three months, the surgeon removes the ileostomy. The pouch then begins to function as a rectum, and the person no longer needs the ileostomy bag.

# Treatment of Anal Crohn's Disease

Because Crohn's disease can attack the small intestine as well as the colon, the pouch is not used for Crohn's disease. When surgeons tried the pouch for Crohn's disease, the complication rate was very high. In most cases, the Crohn's disease attacked the pouch and it could no longer be used. For those with Crohn's disease, if the colon is very diseased but the rectum is not, then the colon can be removed except for the rectum, and the small intestine can be connected directly to the rectum. In many cases, if the Crohn's disease involving the rectum is not severe, it can be controlled with Rowasa encmas or Rowasa suppositories.

When there is perianal disease associated with Crohn's disease, the antibiotic Flagyl (metronidazole) may help. However, it can cause side effects such as tingling of the nerves and headaches.

A common treatment for fistulas in the anal area due to Crohn's disease is the use of setons. Setons are simply elastic "rubber bands" which are placed through the fistulas. Setons do not cure the fistulas. But, they do prevent pus from accumulating which may also help to reduce pain.

A seton is made of a soft, flexible, elastic strand which does not cause much irritation. In most cases, it it is barely noticable, and does not interfere with daily activities or sexual intercourse. Some patients prefer to use setons for years rather than have their rectum removed.

If there are severe fistulas in the anorectal area, the rectum may need to be removed. The person must then learn to get along with either a colostomy or ileostomy bag.

# Stomas

Sometimes surgeons must bring a portion of the intestine through the abdominal muscles out to the skin. This is called an "ileostomy" if the small intestine is used and "colostomy" if the colon is used. The intestinal contents come out through the opening of the skin (stoma) and are collected in a bag worn on the surface of the body.

Fortunately, with today's techniques a permanent stoma is only necessary if the anal sphincters are permanently damaged by, for example, cancer, infection or inflammation.

# Proctitis

Proctitis is an inflammation of the rectum that looks just like ulcerative colitis but does not extend above 10 inches. Proctitis, even though it looks like ulcerative colitis, is much different because 90% of those who have proctitis never develop colitis higher up in the colon. In the majority of people with proctitis, the disease responds rapidly to medications and does not recur.

Proctitis is treated with Rowasa enemas, Rowasa suppositories, Cort enemas, or with Azulfidine or Prednisone by mouth. A much less expensive treatment for proctitis is a mixture of hydrocortisone and Safflower oil. The pharmacist mixes this, and the patient takes it as an enema once or twice a day.

The condition continues to recur and requires periodic treatment in about 10% of proctitis patients.

## *Radiation Proctitis*

Radiation proctitis is a form of proctitis which is caused by radiation therapy. Radiation therapy is generally given for cancer of the prostate or female organs. It can cause a burn on the lining of the rectum. Radiation proctitis does not respond as well as ulcerative proctitis to the use of enemas and suppositories.

Sometimes severe bleeding can occur with radiation proctitis. If enemas and suppositories do not help, and the bleeding becomes severe, topical chemicals such as formalin may stop the bleeding. Surgery may be required to remove the rectum.

# Diverticulosis and Related Conditions

## Diverticulosis

Diverticuli are small sacs or pouches on the wall of the colon. They are similar to the small bulge that appears on a rubber inner tube tire. This condition is known as diverticulosis. The sacs are caused by high pressures within the colon which occur when there is not enough fiber in the bowel movement (feces).

When the colon is relatively empty, normal contractions of the colon muscles cause very high pressures in isolated segments that are empty. These high pressures cause bulging to occur in certain weak spots of the colon, where blood vessels enter the wall from the outside. These sacs, or diverticuli, can get as large as 1/2 inch in size.

Diverticuli do not empty well. Feces can be trapped in these sacs and then become infected, causing inflammation. This causes pain, irritation and scarring. Scarring may cause adhesions later which may twist (kink) the colon.

## Diverticulitis

Diverticulitis is an inflammation of the little sacs (pouches) due to infection. It causes pain or tenderness to the touch. Doctors give antibiotics by vein in the hospital if the pain, tenderness and swelling are severe. Swelling can cause blockage of the colon. Infected diverticuli can rupture. Such a condition requires surgery.

In about 95% of cases, the diverticuli do not cause any symptoms. Diverticuli are very common; perhaps 50% of people over age 60 have diverticuli.

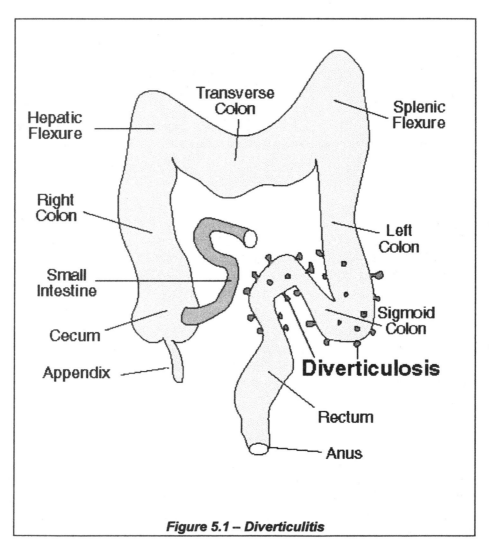

**Figure 5.1 – Diverticulitis**

## Surgery for Diverticulosis

Doctors recommend surgery after two attacks of diverticulitis requiring hospitalization with intravenous antibiotics. The operation is done through an abdominal incision and 12 to 18 inches of the colon are removed.

Less common complications of the diverticulosis are perforation (rupture) of the colon, blockage, and bleeding. If medicines do not cure these complications, then sometimes part of the colon must be removed.

Since diverticuli do not occur in the rectum, it is unusual to need a permanent colostomy for diverticulosis or its complications. With new techniques, surgeons can often avoid even a temporary colostomy. Special techniques clean out the colon during surgery so that even emergency surgery does not require a colostomy as it did in the early 1990s.

## Diarrhea After Gallbladder Surgery

Some people get diarrhea after their gallbladders are removed. This happens in about 1 case in 20 (5% of the time). This is due to irritation of the colon and intestines by the bile salts produced by the liver which can no longer be stored in the gallbladder. People with this problem need to move their bowels immediately after eating or they have multiple, frequent, liquid bowel movements.

This can be easily treated with a medicine called Questran (cholestyramine), which binds to the bile salts and prevents them from irritating the colon.

## Coccygodynia

Coccygodynia is pain in the tailbone due to inflammation. The pain is at the joint where the tail bone (coccyx) connects with the bottom of the spine (sacrum). Injection of a steroid and a pain killer into the joint may cure it. This is done in the physician's office. In severe cases the surgeon removes the tail bone.

## Proctalgia

Proctalgia is pain due to spasm or "Charlie horse" of the pelvic floor muscles, the muscles of the anal sphincter, or the muscles of the rectum. Just as spasms of neck muscles cause headaches, spasms of the pelvic muscles cause proctalgia. This causes severe stabbing pain like a knife sticking into the rectum. It may pass quickly or might last much longer.

Often the pain will awaken the person at night out of a sound sleep. If the person gets up and walks around, moves his bowels, or passes gas, the pain will resolve in a matter of minutes. Some people have spasms of these muscles which lasts continuously through the day and for many weeks at a time. Proctalgia can be related to stress.

There are several treatments for proctalgia. The first is natural vegetable powder in a dose of three heaping tablespoonfuls per day. With this dose, a person should have large, soft bowel movements that stretch out the muscles and help prevent muscle spasms.

If this does not work, muscle relaxants such as Diazepam can be used to relax the muscles.

Pelvic muscle retraining may also be helpful. If *voluntary* muscles are in spasm, a person can be trained to relax these muscles by doing special exercises.

Another possible treatment is electrical stimulation. A small probe about the size of person's finger is inserted into the anal canal. A low voltage vibrating current is passed through the spastic muscles for approximately thirty minutes for each treatment. This may cause the muscles that are in spasm to relax.

Epidural nerve blocks help some people. For this treatment, an anesthesiologist puts a small needle into the person's back and injects a numbing solution, similar to Novocain, which numbs the nerves in the pelvic area.

The muscles of the rectum are not under voluntary control, and cannot be trained to relax. Medicines such as Levsinex SL may relieve *involuntary* rectal muscle spasm.

# Polyps

Polyps are small growths on the inner colon lining that look like warts. It is not known exactly how polyps form, but it has to do with changes that occur as the old lining gets rubbed off and new lining grows. Polyps will form if the old lining does not rub off quickly enough, or if the new lining grows too fast. Genetic changes in cells cause normal colon lining to turn into polyps.

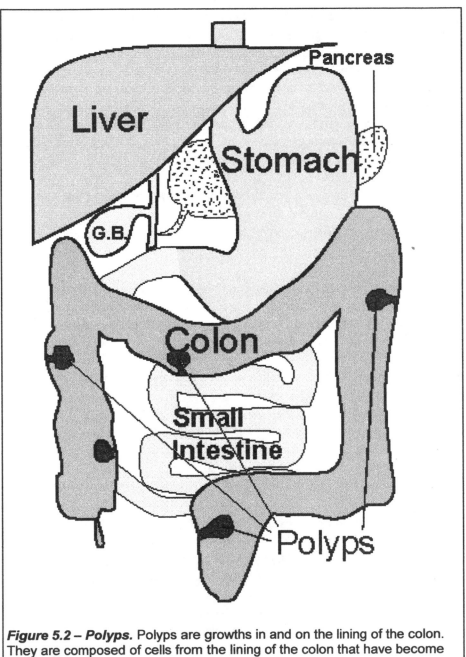

***Figure 5.2 – Polyps.*** Polyps are growths in and on the lining of the colon. They are composed of cells from the lining of the colon that have become genetically altered.

When the cells that make up the lining of the colon are in their genetically altered state they no longer conform to the usual rules that govern them. These rules include: stand up straight beside one another, don't cluster together in unruly mobs, disappear when you're supposed to and definitely don't go running around to other parts of the body. If the cells of the lining of the colon don't follow these rules then they form polyps. If polyps remain, the cells keeping the "bad company" get increasingly unruly and eventually can turn into invasive cancers. These invasive cancers can then eat through the wall of the colon or they can spread to other parts of the body as metastases.

Sometimes the body may eradicate polyps, or polyps may be removed by a doctor. Removing colon polyps can prevent colon cancer. Polyps are removed through a colonoscope without the need for surgery.

## Types of Polyps

The only way to determine what kind of polyp a patient has is to remove the polyp and examine it under a microscope. An *inflammatory polyp* forms in reaction to ulceration or irritation. Inflammatory polyps are often seen in cases of colitis. They will not turn into cancer.

*Hyperplastic polyps* also have a very low risk of turning into cancer. *Adenomatous polyps* may eventually become cancerous. A person with adenomatous polyps should have repeat colonoscopies every three years to look for, and remove, new polyps.

A *villous polyp* is aggressive and more likely to turn into cancer. Villous polyps should be removed completely when they are found. They require a colonoscopy one year after they are removed, and every one to three years after that. Sometimes they are so large that they must be removed with surgery.

A few people develop many, many – hundreds, even thousands of polyps – in their colons. This is called *polyposis coli*. This condition tends to run in families. If a mother or father has polyposis coli, chances are that half their children will have it. If these polyps are not treated and removed, nearly all individuals with this condition will develop cancer of the colon or rectum by the time they are 40 years old. The treatment for polyposis coli is removal of the colon and creation of a new rectum using the small intestine.

# 6

# Constipation:
# The Last Taboo

Nobody wants to talk about the "C" word, *constipation*. People can talk about unusual sexual acts on mid-afternoon television but no one will talk about constipation. In our society it is impolite to talk about one's bowel function. This means many people with constipation and its relatives, bloating, abdominal pain, straining, rectal pain and pelvic pressure, suffer in silence. They are embarrassed to mention it to friends, family and even physicians. If they do mention bowel trouble to their doctor they are usually put off with instructions to eat more salads and fiber. However, it is not really their physician's fault. Most doctors receive little or no education on constipation during medical school, internship or residency.

## What is Constipation?

Constipation is difficult, painful, or infrequent bowel movements. The normal frequency of bowel movements is from three times per day to three times per week. Usually, if more than three days pass between bowel movements, the intestinal contents harden. Hard stools are difficult and painful to pass.

Doctors define constipation as:

- Less than 3 bowel movements per week.
- Having to strain to move your bowels more than 25% of the time.
- Having painful bowel movements more than 25% of the time.
- Having to use your fingers or hands to help move your bowels.

It is not necessary to move your bowels every day. Even if the waste products stay in the intestines for longer than three days, they will not harm the body or cause cancer.

## How Common is Constipation?

As little as people talk about constipation one would think that no one suffers from it. Yet, nothing is further from the truth! Constipation is very common. According to medical studies (Drossman in *Digestive Diseases and Sciences*, September, 1993), 3% of the nation's population suffer from constipation.

To put this in perspective, this means that 6,000 people in Charleston County, South Carolina – where this author's practice is located – (population: about 200,000) suffer from constipation. According to this same study, 32% of the nation's population suffer from abdominal bloating. This translates to 64,000 people in Charleston County. Moreover, nearly 2%, 3,400 in Charleston County, suffer from chronic abdominal pain; 11%, 22,000 people in Charleston County, suffer from anal or rectal pain; and 13%, 27,000 in Charleston County, suffer from difficult rectal emptying.

### Who should be evaluated for constipation?

Ingesting 25-30 grams of fiber daily corrects 90-95% of symptoms of constipation. Any time that constipation does not respond to increased fiber and the constipation interferes with sleep, work or the enjoyment of life, it warrants further evaluation.

## Causes of Constipation

Causes of constipation can be broken down into two groups: 1) problems outside of the colon that effect the colon and 2) problems with the colon, rectum and anus.

### Causes outside the colon

- *Low Fiber Diet* – The most common cause of constipation is a lack of fiber in the diet. This can be corrected by ingesting 25-30 grams of fiber daily. A balanced diet along with a supplement such as three heaping tablespoons of Natural Vegetable Powder in a glass of juice, milk or water daily will ensure this amount of fiber.

- *Poor Bowel Habits* – If a person frequently ignores the urge to move his bowels, the rectum and colon can get stretched out. If this happens often, it may become harder and harder for the rectum to sense when it is full. This may cause constipation.

- *Glandular or Hormonal Problems* – Constipation can be caused by hormonal problems such as thyroid disease.

- *Medication* – Medicines can cause constipation. Pain medications, especially narcotics, antacids that contain aluminum, antispasm drugs, anticonvulsants (for epilepsy), tranquilizers, antidepressants, and iron supplements can all cause constipation.

- *Pregnancy* – Hormonal changes and the weight of the full womb during pregnancy can cause constipation.

- *Nerve damage* – Spinal cord injuries, spinal cord tumors, and nerve diseases can cause constipation.

- *Medical Illnesses* – When people are sick their bowels may not work well. Diabetes, scleroderma, neurological diseases like Parkinson's disease, and multiple sclerosis and other medical illnesses can affect the intestines and cause constipation.

## Colon, Rectum and Anus Problems

### Colon Blockage

Narrowing of the colon can make it hard for waste (feces) to pass. Inflammation, diverticulitis, scar tissue, large polyps, and cancer can all cause narrowing, or partial blockage, of the colon. These causes are not very common. A barium enema or colonoscopy can show if a blockage exists.

If none of the above problems is present then we look for problems with the *function* of the colon itself. A simple way to understand these problems is to think of the colon as a pump. If the pump pumps too slowly, or if the pump is blocked, then constipation will occur.

Some other treatable causes of constipation are:

1) Slow transit or colonic inertia
2) Rectal descent
3) Rectocele

4) Tight internal sphincter
5) Non-relaxing puborectalis
6) Cecal bascule

## Slow Colon (Colonic Inertia)

Some people suffer from severe constipation because their colon holds on to feces too long. These people suffer from abdominal pain, "gas," abdominal distention, and bloating. They generally do not complain of difficulty emptying their rectum. Instead, they feel as if their intestinal contents never get to their rectum. If there is nothing else found to be the cause of their symptoms, these people may suffer from colonic inertia, a colon that pumps too slowly.

We confirm the diagnosis with a "transit time" measurement that tells us how fast the colon works. We describe this test later. We must also rule out any other cause of slow colon transit such as low thyroid hormone levels.

If the colon works too slowly and the person suffers from constipation with abdominal pain and bloating which make daily activities difficult, then surgery may be needed. Surgically shortening the colon corrects a slow colon. Most of the colon is removed, and the small intestine is attached directly to the rectum. This procedure does *not* require a colostomy (a new opening of the colon onto the abdominal skin requiring a bag).

How many constipated people need this operation? Between May, 1991, and December, 1994, I treated 4,500 people with colon and rectal complaints. Of these, 778 people had constipation. Of these 778 constipated people, only 31 needed their colons surgically shortened.

# Surgery for Colonic Inertia

Colon surgery will relieve constipation due to slow colonic transit in nearly all patients. The surgery will substantially relieve pain in over two-thirds of these patients.

The surgery for slow colon is considered major surgery. It is not quite as dangerous as open heart surgery, chest or brain surgery, but it is major surgery. It is a bigger operation than a hysterectomy. It involves removing about 80% of the large intestine. The technical term for the operation is "total abdominal colectomy and ileorectal anastomosis."

There are several steps. First, we enter the abdomen by making an up and down cut from two inches above the belly button (umbilicus), around the belly button and then down to the top of the pelvic bone (pubis).

The second step is mobilizing (freeing up) the colon. The large intestine (colon) is attached to the muscles of the back by a filmy, strong tissue. We divide the strong film so that we can pull the colon away from the back muscles.

When we mobilize the colon we are careful not to injure organs behind the colon, like the duodenum (first part of the small intestine), the pancreas (which makes digestive juices and insulin), the spleen (which filters the blood), and the ureters (which carry urine from the kidneys to the bladder).

Now the colon is still attached to the small intestine at one end and the rectum at the other, and to an arcade, or net, of blood vessels. These blood vessels start out as three main trunks, then branch into a dozen or so branches. These branches then branch again into hundreds of small blood vessels that go into the colon to carry blood to and from the colon.

After we have freed up the colon, we can see the blood vessels clearly. We clamp, cut and tie off each of the blood vessel branches except those going to the rectum (the last part of the colon).

We clamp the ileum (last part of the small intestine), where it attaches to the colon, and cut it between two clamps. The clamps keep anything in the colon and ileum, such as mucus, from spilling out during the procedure.

Now the colon is attached only to the rectum. The top of the rectum is closed off with a straight stapler placing a double row of staples across the top of the rectum. The colon is then cut just above the staple line and removed from the body. The ileum is then attached to the rectum with a special stapling instrument that places two circular rows of staples.

After attaching the ileum to the rectum, we check the anastomosis (connection) by squirting air and iodine solution into the rectum to make sure that the anastomosis is water and air tight. We check for bleeding. Then we close the abdomen and the skin with sutures.

When the surgery is completed, the patient is transferred to the recovery room and then to a hospital room for recuperation. The patient does not eat for three to five days, but receives water and calories by vein. A nurse assists the patient in walking several times each day. A tube in the bladder empties urine for a few days.

The bowels usually start working three to five days after surgery, but sometimes it takes longer. The patient will start taking liquids four or five days after the surgery. If there are no complications, the person goes home in five to nine days.

It is best to stay on a full liquid diet, including puddings, soups and ice creams, for two more days at home. After surgery, patients should eat food in small amounts and chew it thoroughly. There may be cramps and gas pains for a while. Usually most of the cramps and gas pains will be gone within three months.

Liquid bowel movements are common for the first few weeks or months after the surgery. For the first month or two, the bowels may move six to ten times per day. On the average, most people move their bowels three times each day as the final result. Until the patient is accustomed to the new "plumbing" and softer stool, some "accidents" or leakage will occur. Usually these accidents do not last long. If the bowels are moving too often, medications can be used to slow them down.

In the weeks before the surgery, patients may donate one or two units of their own blood. Then, if blood is needed during the operation or recovery period, the individual gets his own blood back. For two days prior to surgery, the person takes oral laxatives and antibiotics to clean the colon.

As with any major surgery, there are risks and potential complications. After the surgery, there may be internal bleeding and blood transfusions may be necessary. Sometimes, reoperation to control bleeding is necessary. Infection can occur inside the abdomen requiring antibiotics or drainage. Scar tissue can form inside the abdomen that can kink the small intestine, causing blockage. Sometimes, this must be treated with surgery to cut the scar tissue to release the blockage. In our experience, about four cases in forty needed surgery for scar tissue (adhesions) causing blockage.

The anastomosis where the ileum is hooked to the rectum can scar and narrow, requiring dilatation with a balloon through the rectum. The anastomosis can leak causing infection, and possibly the need for further surgery. Fortunately, this is uncommon. There is little risk of an ileostomy or a colostomy being necessary for this surgery. If one were required, it is usually only temporary. So far, we have not done one in 50 people having this surgery.

About 1 person in 100 may have trouble with their lungs after surgery. They may have trouble breathing and need to be on a mechanical ventilator while their lungs improve. Smoking increases the risk of lung problems after surgery. Even if people do not smoke, they can have trouble with their lungs after surgery. Anytime that you have general anesthesia (you are put to sleep for surgery) there is some risk to your life. This risk is very small especially if you are less than 60 years old, and do not have heart or lung disease. If you are over 60, (we have done this on people as old as 73), or have heart or lung disease, you can still have the surgery, but the risks are higher.

## Rectal Descent

Some people have great difficulty emptying their rectum due to what is called rectal descent. Rectal descent is a problem that appears to be related to childbirth. When a women gives birth, the normal attachments of the rectum to the lower backbone may get stretched or torn. This tearing allows the rectum to fall into the pelvis where it assumes a horizontal position. The front of the rectum can fall into the top of the anal canal and block the anal opening.

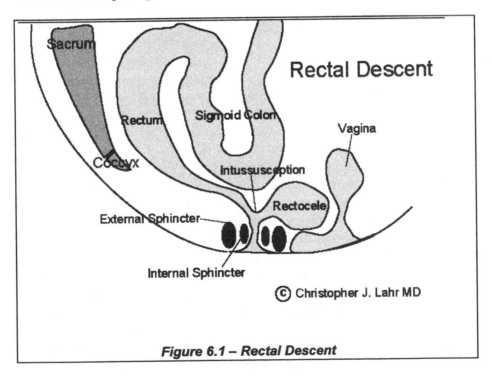

**Figure 6.1 – Rectal Descent**

The normal rectum lies against the sacrum (lower backbone) in a gentle curve down to the anal opening. When a person moves his bowels, the muscles of the pelvic floor relax and the rectum swings down and straightens

*Shining Light on Constipation*

so it is almost straight up and down (vertical) over the anal opening. In this way the rectal contents can move straight out. (See Figure 6.2.)

When a person pushes to move his or her bowels, it increases abdominal pressure. If the rectum is attached to the sacrum properly, the increased abdominal pressure squeezes the rectal contents out like toothpaste from a tube. The rectum is a soft pliable tube. If it is not firmly supported by the lower backbone, it slides down in the pelvis and blocks the anal opening.

Let us compare the rectum to a sock. If you support the sock with one hand on either side of the top open end, then it is easy to put your foot into it and slide it all the way inside. If, however, the sock is lying on the floor not supported or held in place, then it will be very hard to put your foot into it, much less get your foot all of the way in. The same is true of the rectum. The hands supporting the sock are represented by the attachments of the top of the rectum to the backbone.

Another comparison might be to a pair of pants. They are easy to put on if you lift them up with your hands on the waistline. It is more difficult to put them on if they are lying crumpled on the floor and you can't grab the waist band with your hands. It is easier to push something through a soft pliable tube if it is supported at the top and hanging vertically then if it is lying flat horizontally.

Knowing this, you can predict the complaints that people with rectal descent have. If they don't have colonic inertia, they will have the usual amounts of stool getting down to the rectum daily. They will feel the urge to move their bowels; but, even with straining, the rectum will not empty. This differs from someone with colonic inertia. Someone with colonic inertia may not feel the need to move his bowels for a week or more at a time. Someone with rectal descent without colonic inertia will feel the need to move his bowels every day.

It takes people with rectal descent a long time to move their bowels. They may try to move their bowels several times before they are able to. Even after they move their bowels, it may feel as if their rectum is still not empty.

They may feel a mass pushing against their vagina or they may feel as if their rectum is dropping out of their pelvis. They may feel a weight down on the bottom of their pelvis.

People with rectal descent have difficulty emptying their rectum. They must strain to move their bowels. They may have to put their fingers into their rectum or vagina, or push on their pelvic area, to get their bowels to move.

When we operate on people with rectal descent we sometimes see that the rectum has fallen down into the pelvis and is just lying flat on the floor of the pelvis. Before talking about how to correct rectal descent let us discuss some other forms of rectal descent. The first is solitary rectal ulcer.

## Solitary Rectal Ulcer

Sometimes rectal descent causes the front wall of the rectum to flop into the anal canal (see Figure 6.1). Straining causes pressure on the front wall of the rectum and a pressure sore develops. This sore is called a solitary rectal ulcer. It has a white base and sharp distinct edges. When we see it, we can be certain that rectal descent is present. This solitary rectal ulcer can cause pain and bleeding. One person bled so much from her solitary rectal ulcer that she needed to receive seven units of blood. This can also occur in males.

## Rectocele

Rectocele is a bulge of the lower rectum into, over or behind the vagina. Rectoceles trap stool and may not empty. Rectoceles are probably more common in women after hysterectomy. The rectum falls into the place of the uterus. The woman with a rectocele may need to put her finger into the vagina to push the stool out. Defecography demonstrates the rectum bulging forward. Stool softeners and fiber may help. If they do not, surgery may be needed.

I believe that rectoceles are a form of rectal descent. They can only occur if the attachments between the rectum and the vagina are weakened, and if extra rectum is dragged down or stretched out to form the pouch.

If the rectocele causes difficult rectal emptying, I believe that the associated rectal descent must be corrected. The surgery recommended for a symptomatic rectocele is the same operation done for rectal descent

A type of rectocele repair can be done through the vagina, but this does not correct rectal descent. It often does not correct the rectal emptying problems associated with rectoceles.

We can usually confirm that a woman has rectal descent by talking to her and examining her. We must confirm the diagnosis with defecography. Defecography uses video X-rays to look at the shape and position of the rectum as it empties. We describe this test later.

## *Surgery for Rectal Descent*

Rectal descent is a physical, mechanical problem. If medical treatment fails, it can be corrected with surgery. However, having rectal descent is not like having a cancer. People don't die from rectal descent; therefore, they don't need to have surgery unless they want it.

The requirements for considering surgery for rectal descent are:

- The person has symptoms of rectal descent.

- Signs of rectal descent are seen on defecography (X-ray).

- Difficult rectal emptying interferes with the ability to enjoy life and to work productively.

- The person wishes to have surgery.

- Other medical problems (such as heart or lung disease) do not make the risk of surgery so high that risks outweigh possible benefits.

The surgery for rectal descent has three parts: 1) The colon is shortened by removing the sigmoid colon (sigmoid resection); 2) The sides of the rectum are lifted up and sewn with suspender stitches to the lower backbone (rectopexy); 3) The space between the rectum and vagina is closed to support the rectum and to prevent the intestines from filling this sapce. Finally we may also add a piece of Goretex (like they use to make gloves), to support the weight of the rectum and vagina.

Removing the sigmoid colon involves cutting out about 8 to 12 inches of colon just above the rectum. This is called the sigmoid colon because it is shaped like an "S." In people with rectal descent, the sigmoid colon has a tendency to fall down in the pelvis. Removing it (and hooking the ends together) straightens the left side of the colon. This makes it easier for stool to pass. Since the sigmoid colon is removed, it cannot flop over the rectopexy stitches causing a kink in the rectum.

Lateral stalks of fibrous tissue support the rectum on either side. A soft strong suture of Goretex is used to pass a stitch through the lateral stalk on one side of the rectum. Then it is passed through the surface of the sacrum (lower backbone). This is repeated three times. When these sutures are tied they pull the rectum up and attach it firmly again to the top of the sacrum. This is the rectopexy.

If there is a deep space between the rectum and the vagina that allows the intestines to fall down into or through the pelvic floor (enterocele) then we close this space by putting three rows of sutures in the front wall of the rectum and the back wall of the vagina. With each suture, several running stitches are made. When all three rows of stitches are in place, they are tied gently and not too tightly, so that they pull the front of the rectum together with the back of the vagina.

Finally, a piece of Goretex is sewn to the rectopexy stitches and then to the top of the vagina. When the knots on the Goretex patch are tied the weight of the front of the rectum and the vagina rests on the backbone. It no longer rests on the muscles of the pelvic floor. In lifting up the vagina we are also attempting to straighten out the front of the rectum so that it no longer bulges forward (rectocele).

The post-operative recovery is very similar to that after colon resection for colonic inertia (slow colon). The risks and possible complications are about the same.

## Rectal Prolapse

Another form of rectal descent is rectal prolapse. When the rectum falls down in the pelvis it can drop so far that it actually drops through the anal opening as a pink fleshy round lump. This is called rectal prolapse. Rectal prolapse can block the anal opening causing constipation. The prolapse can stretch the anal sphincter muscles and cause anal leakage (incontinence).

Rectal prolapse is not a cancer and it will not turn into a cancer. Therefore, treatment is necessary only if it is causing a problem.

Symptoms of prolapse which might indicate the need for surgery include persistent bleeding, chronic constipation, difficulty with rectal emptying, straining to move the bowels, mucous drainage, protruding lump, inability to control solid, liquid, or gas bowel movements, or progressive weakening of the anal sphincter muscles.

The aim of the surgery is to remove the extra rectal length and re-suspend the rectum from the lower backbone.

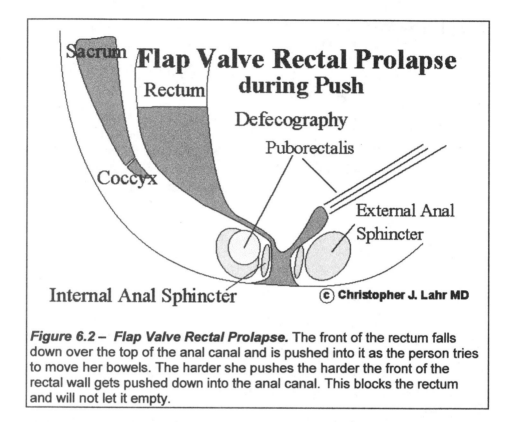

**Figure 6.2 – Flap Valve Rectal Prolapse.** The front of the rectum falls down over the top of the anal canal and is pushed into it as the person tries to move her bowels. The harder she pushes the harder the front of the rectal wall gets pushed down into the anal canal. This blocks the rectum and will not let it empty.

Prolapse can be repaired by either anal surgery or abdominal surgery. In the abdominal surgery, the sigmoid colon is removed and the rectum is sewn to the sacrum (just like the surgery for rectal descent).

Another way to accomplish bowel shortening and re-suspension is to remove the extra rectal length through the anus. Then, the bowel ends are hooked together just above the anus. Removing all the excess bowel leaves the shortened rectum hanging from the inside of the abdomen on the left, by the spleen and ribs. This operation does not require an incision on the front of the abdomen and there is no risk of damage to the nerves of the penis in men.

If a person has rectal prolapse and fecal incontinence (the inability to control bowel movements), fixing the rectal prolapse about half the time also corrects the incontinence. However, if the sphincter muscles are very weak, fixing the prolapse will not correct the incontinence. Additional surgery may be needed to tighten the anal sphincter muscles.

# Anal Stenosis

Two muscles make up the anal sphincters: an *internal* and an *external* anal sphincter. The internal anal sphincter is a thin, white muscle wrapped around the anal canal. The internal sphincter contracts during rest and sleep, and keeps small amounts of liquid and gas from escaping unexpectedly. The internal anal sphincter is involuntary smooth muscle, like the muscles of your intestines. One cannot control it mentally.

The external anal sphincter is a thick, red voluntary muscle. It is wrapped around the internal anal sphincter muscle. It is the one you squeeze when you feel the urge to go to the bathroom but are not near one. Since it is voluntary muscle, like the muscles in your arms and legs, you can control it.

Anal stenosis means that the anal opening is too small, or that it does not relax or open properly. Scar tissue can cause anal stenosis. This may need to be treated with surgery that brings a flap of skin down to enlarge the anal opening.

In some people, the internal anal sphincter does not relax as it should. This makes the anal opening too small. If it causes severe constipation or painful and difficult rectal emptying, a tight internal anal sphincter can be treated with dilatation or with a surgical myotomy (cutting the muscle).

# Non-relaxing Puborectalis

At the bottom of the rectum, just as it is about to go into the anal canal, the rectum is kinked by the puborectalis muscle. The puborectalis muscle starts at the pubic bone, loops around the bottom of the rectum, and returns to the pubic bone like a sling.

The puborectalis is a voluntary muscle. Puborectalis contraction kinks the lower rectum so rectal contents are not expelled when abdominal pressure increases.

When coughing or lifting something heavy the puborectalis and external sphincter muscles tighten to prevent rectal contents from being pushed out.

The nerve supply to these two muscles is very similar. They contract together, unless one muscle has been injured or cut. The puborectalis and external anal sphincter must relax to let the rectum empty. If the external sphincter and puborectalis tighten during straining then it is harder for the rectum to empty. We call this non-relaxing puborectalis, paradoxical puborectalis, spastic pelvic floor or anismus.

Since these are voluntary muscles, they can sometimes be retrained just as a bad golf swing can be corrected through retraining and practice. To improve muscle function, the person must be able to see what his muscles are doing. We use computer equipment that shows the person how his sphincter muscles are moving. We call this treatment pelvic muscle retraining. It can also be used to strengthen weak muscles as we will discuss later.

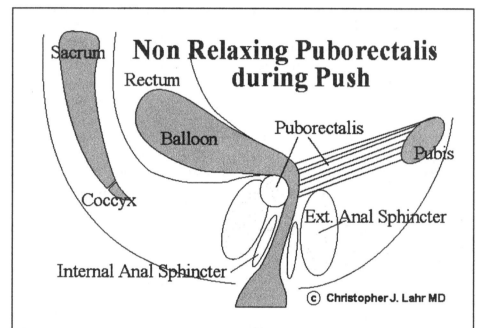

**Non Relaxing Puborectalis during Push**

Sacrum
Rectum
Balloon
Coccyx
Puborectalis
Pubis
Ext. Anal Sphincter
Internal Anal Sphincter

© Christopher J. Lahr MD

*Figure 6.3 – Non-Relaxing Puborectalis/Pelvic Diaphragm.* Side view. This is an inappropriate learned response. Some people feel that to move their bowels they must markedly increase their intraabdominal pressure. To do this, they tighten their pelvic diaphragm. This allows them to increase their intraabdominal pressure, but it also increases the kink in their lower rectum. Since the external anal sphincter usually contracts with the pelvic diaphragm, the anal canal is also closed. This makes it very difficult for the person to move his bowels. The harder he tries to push, the tighter the pelvic diaphragm and the external anal sphincter get. Since the pelvic diaphragm muscles and the external anal sphincter muscle are voluntary muscles, this inappropriate response can be corrected with pelvic muscle retraining.

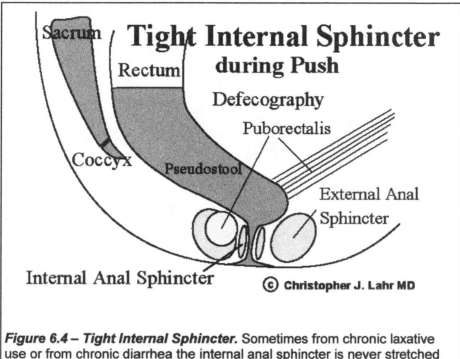

**Figure 6.4 – Tight Internal Sphincter.** Sometimes from chronic laxative use or from chronic diarrhea the internal anal sphincter is never stretched out and it becomes too tight and will not stretch out as it should to open the anal canal. Just as muscles at the elbow joint can form contractures if the elbow is in a cast for a long time, the internal anal sphincter can tighten up so it will not open. The internal anal sphincter muscle is not a voluntary muscle that can be readily altered by retraining. Therefore a tight internal anal sphincter must be treated with dilation or with surgical myotomy, which is cutting the muscle.

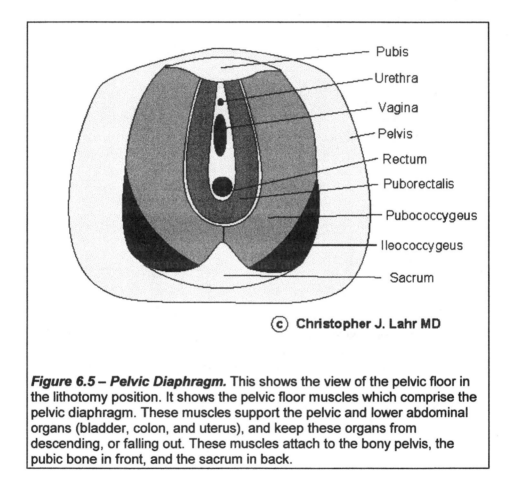

Pubis
Urethra
Vagina
Pelvis
Rectum
Puborectalis
Pubococcygeus
Ileococcygeus
Sacrum

ⓒ Christopher J. Lahr MD

*Figure 6.5 – Pelvic Diaphragm.* This shows the view of the pelvic floor in the lithotomy position. It shows the pelvic floor muscles which comprise the pelvic diaphragm. These muscles support the pelvic and lower abdominal organs (bladder, colon, and uterus), and keep these organs from descending, or falling out. These muscles attach to the bony pelvis, the pubic bone in front, and the sacrum in back.

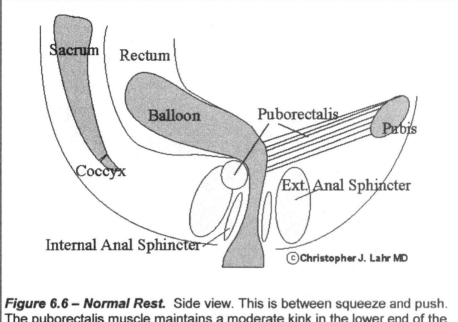

*Figure 6.6 – Normal Rest.* Side view. This is between squeeze and push. The puborectalis muscle maintains a moderate kink in the lower end of the rectum. The internal anal sphincter also maintains a moderate amount of contraction that keeps the anal canal closed. These two mechanisms prevent the escape of gas, liquid and solid stool during rest, sleep, and inactivity.

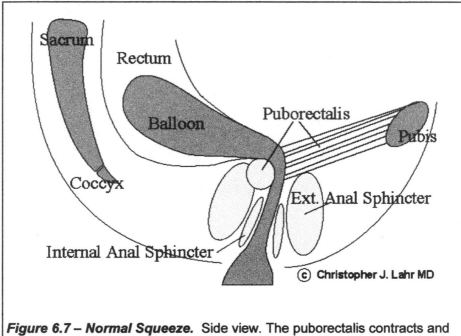

*Figure 6.7 – Normal Squeeze.* Side view. The puborectalis contracts and shortens. This kinks the bottom of the rectum as it enters the anal canal. The external anal sphincter contracts, tightening like a noose around the anal canal. This helps prevent gas, liquid or solid stool from escaping from the rectum during any maneuver that increases intra-abdominal pressure, such as coughing, shouting, or lifting.

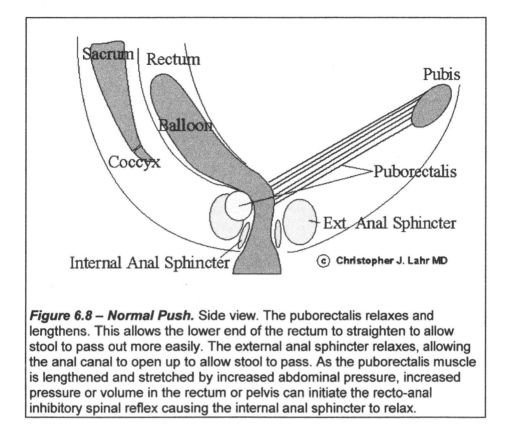

*Figure 6.8 – Normal Push.* Side view. The puborectalis relaxes and lengthens. This allows the lower end of the rectum to straighten to allow stool to pass out more easily. The external anal sphincter relaxes, allowing the anal canal to open up to allow stool to pass. As the puborectalis muscle is lengthened and stretched by increased abdominal pressure, increased pressure or volume in the rectum or pelvis can initiate the recto-anal inhibitory spinal reflex causing the internal anal sphincter to relax.

## Cecal Bascule

The colon is ordinarily attached to the muscles of the back by thin, but strong attachments. These prevent the colon from moving around inside of the abdominal cavity. If these attachments are too long, the colon can swing freely inside the abdominal cavity.

The cecum is the part of the right colon that attaches to the small intestine. When the cecum can swing freely inside the abdomen, it is called a cecal bascule. Bascule is the French word for a draw bridge that raises up on one side and is hinged on the other. The point where the colon is hinged can kink, blocking the colon. The part of the colon that swings can become filled with stool or waste. It gets stretched out because it can not empty past the kinked portion. This stretching causes pain and bloating.

People with a cecal bascule will complain of severe intermittent abdominal pain, constipation, and bloating. They will not have any trouble emptying their rectum once the stool gets there. They usually move their bowels with normal frequency, although they may miss some days when they are having pain. Then, they have diarrhea or explosive stools when the cecum becomes unkinked and suddenly releases pent-up stool. This relieves the pain. Their transit times are normal.

Cecal bascule is generally seen on barium enema. This is treated by removing the free-floating part of the colon and hooking the ends back together.

Cecal bascule and tight internal sphincter are not as common as slow colon and rectal descent.

# Special Tests for Constipation

Either a colonoscopy or an air-contrast barium enema and sigmoidoscopy is required in people with constipation to rule out obstruction, polyps, inflammatory bowel disease, diverticulosis and stricture.
If none of these problems are found, we will look for another cause of constipation by doing the tests that we call a constipation diagnostic panel including:

1) Transit time
2) Defecography
3) Sphincterography
4) Anorectal manometry
5) Pudendal nerve study
6) Anal sphincter electromyography

These tests can be done on the same day. It takes about five hours to complete. They can be divided and done on two days.

# Transit Time Measurement

A transit time X-ray measures the time it takes for food to go through the colon. The person takes special capsules by mouth twice a day for five days. Each capsule has 12 X-ray markers. Each day, the person takes a total of 24 markers. This averages out to one every hour.

On the sixth day, an X-ray of the abdomen is taken and we count the number of markers left in the person's colon. This tells about how long it takes for food to go through the colon. If there are 86 markers, it takes 86 hours. If there are only 24 markers, it takes 24 hours.

The average normal transit time is 35 hours. The upper limit of normal is 72 hours. If it takes more than 72 hours to go through the body, and all other tests are normal, then we make the diagnosis of colonic inertia (slow transit).

It is important to avoid the use of **all** laxatives and enemas during the five days before a transit time X-ray. However, it is fine to continue natural vegetable powder, or other fiber supplements, in a normal dose.

# Sphincterography

Sphincterography is an X-ray to evaluate voluntary muscle strength and relaxation. Sphincterography uses a flexible balloon connected to a bag of liquid barium. The pressure inside the balloon is equal to the height of the barium bag above the balloon. The higher the bag, the higher the balloon pressure.

The person lies on his left side and a deflated balloon is inserted into the anal canal and rectum. Barium fills the balloon. X-rays are taken while the person squeezes, relaxes, and pushes. These X-rays tell how strong the sphincter is and if it relaxes properly.

# Defecography

Defecography uses X-ray to look at the shape and postion of the rectum as it empties. The anal canal is lubricated and a soft plastic tip is inserted through the anal canal into the rectum. The rectum and anal canal are filled with barium paste and the tip is removed.

X-ray dye is placed in the urinary bladder and the vagina. The person drinks barium about one hour before the test so the small intestine shows up. This way everything in the pelvis can be seen when the person strains.

The person sits on a toilet-like seat, called a defecography chair, which is attached to the X-ray table. The table is tilted into the upright position. The person puts their elbows on their knees. The person is asked to squeeze, to push and to empty the rectum. The X-ray of these maneuvers is recorded on videotape.

Defecography shows the rectum as it empties. Defecography reveals rectoceles and signs of rectal descent. In women with rectal descent, there is more rectal length down in the bottom 3 inches of the pelvis.

A normal rectum should empty in just a few seconds. In rectal descent it may take 30, 60 or even 90 seconds to empty, and the rectum may not empty completely. The lower end of the rectum may close before the upper rectum is empty (flap valving).

People with a tight internal anal sphincter have a big bowl-shaped rectum that empties slowly through a narrow, short anal opening that never opens up.

People with non-relaxing puborectalis muscles have rectums that do not empty because the pelvic floor muscles do not relax.

Defecography findings of rectal descent are:

• Rectocele
• Horizontal rectum during push
• Delayed or incomplete rectal emptying
• Delayed or incomplete rectocele emptying
• Rectum protruding into anal canal
• Long rectum in the bottom 3 inches of the pelvis

## Ano-Rectal Manometry

Ano-rectal manometry measures pressures of the anal sphincter muscles. It also measures how well a person feels different sensations of fullness in the rectum.

A person prepares for the test by using a plain Bisacodyl or Saline enema (for example, Fleets brand) about two to four hours before the test. The enema can be purchased at the drugstore without a prescription. It is important not to eat anything, or drink liquids with caffeine, for about four hours prior to the test.

The person lies on his left side. A small, flexible tube, about the size of a thermometer, is inserted into the rectum. A tiny amount of water drips into the tube while it is connected to a machine that measures pressure.

During the test the nurse asks the person to squeeze, relax, and push. The anal sphincter muscle pressures are measured during each of these maneuvers. To squeeze, the person tightens the sphincter muscles as if trying to prevent anything from coming out. To push, the person strains down as if trying to have a bowel movement.

Ordinarily, the sphincter muscle tightens, and the anal canal pressures increase when the person tries to squeeze. When the person stops squeezing, the muscles should relax, and pressures return to baseline.

When the person pushes, as if having a bowel movement, the sphincter muscles should stay relaxed. This will cause the pressures to stay the same as during rest, or to decrease slightly. If the pressures increase during a push, this may be a sign that the sphincter muscles tighten when pushing. This tightness could contribute to constipation.

Sphincterography and anal manometry show how strong the sphincter muscles are and if they relax as they should during rectal emptying.

Weak muscles that still tighten some can be strengthened with special exercise and treatments. Muscles that do not relax with a push can also be retrained. This is called Pelvic Muscle Retraining and is discussed later.

If the muscles are very weak, some constipation operations may be modified. If a person with colonic inertia has weak sphincters, then to prevent incontinence, the colon may not be shortened as much.

## Pudendal Nerve Studies

Pudendal nerve studies evaluate the nerve to the anal sphincter muscles. A nurse or doctor does a rectal exam with a small electrode taped to the index finger. The nerve inside the rectum is stimulated with a low electrical current. Some people do not feel the stimulus. Others feel a slight "buzz." The nerve stimulus should cause the sphincter muscles to contract. A computer measures how long it takes the sphincter to contract after the nerve is stimulated.

If the pudendal nerve is slow, it is less likely that surgical repair of a weak sphincter will be successful.

## Anal Sphincter EMG

Anal sphincter EMG is recorded with a small sponge electrode in the anal canal. The person relaxes, squeezes and pushes. A computer records sphincter muscle electrical activity.

Anal sphincter electromyography confirms the proper muscle contractions during squeeze and muscle relaxation during push. In people with non-relaxing puborectalis, the tracing of electrical activity gets bigger, instead of smaller, during a push.

Normal anal EMG activity with low anal squeeze pressures on manometry may indicate a torn sphincter muscle that could be repaired.

## Why so Many Tests?

These tests of the "constipation diagnostic profile" are all relatively painless. They may be somewhat embarrassing or uncomfortable for some people; but, most people tolerate them extremely well.

With these tests it can be determined if the person has a slow colon, rectal descent, rectocele, non-relaxing puborectalis, tight internal sphincter, weak anal sphincter, or a combination of these.

The reason so many tests are done when considering surgery is to be sure nothing is missed. We want to plan the best surgical procedure so that the symptoms will be corrected after surgery. With these tests and treatments, it is unusual to find someone whose constipation cannot be relieved.

# 7

# Incontinence (Leakage)

F ecal incontinence is the release of someone's rectal contents against their wishes. Half of all people complaining to doctors of diarrhea have incontinence. Incontinence is the most common cause for institutionalizing an elderly person. It ranks above incompetence. It is a nearly insurmountable obstacle in keeping a child in a public school. Up to 3% of women who give birth vaginally have temporary or permanent fecal incontinence. Fecal incontinence is much more debilitating than urinary incontinence.

## Weak Sphincter Incontinence

There are two muscles which make up the anal sphincters, the internal anal sphincter and the external anal sphincter. The internal anal sphincter is a thin white muscle wrapped around the anal canal. The internal sphincter has a resting tightness which keeps small amounts of liquid and gas from escaping unexpectedly during rest and sleep.

The external anal sphincter is a large thick red voluntary muscle. It is the one you squeeze when you feel the urge to go to the bathroom but are not near a bathroom yet. It is a thick muscle that is wrapped around the internal anal sphincter muscle.

You have conscious, voluntary control over the external anal sphincter. You do not have voluntary control over the internal anal sphincter.

If the anal sphincter muscles become weak after having babies or with increasing age, people may have trouble controlling their bowel movements and gas. They may leak gas, liquid feces, or solid feces, which can cause extreme embarrassment. If this condition cannot be corrected through the use of natural vegetable powder, then other treatment is available.

The anal sphincter muscles can be strengthened without surgery through the use of exercises (pelvic muscle retraining).  If this is not successful,  then surgery may be needed to tighten the anal sphincter muscles.

The external anal sphincter muscles are made of the same kind of muscle as those in a person's arms and legs. Special equipment is used to teach the person how to exercise these muscles.  After they learn how to exercise the sphincter muscles correctly, they can do the exercises at home without special equipment.  The exercises must be done regularly for the rest of a person's life.

If exercises do not help,  or if the sphincter muscles have been cut or torn during childbirth or some previous surgery, then surgery can be performed to repair and tighten the muscles.

Before recommending sphincter repair surgery we study the pudendal nerve.  The pudendal nerve is the nerve to the external anal sphincter.  If it is damaged on both sides, then surgery may not help.

## Pelvic Muscle Retraining

Pelvic muscle retraining helps individuals achieve better control of the pelvic floor muscles. It is effective in treating constipation, incontinence and rectal or pelvic pain.  In the process, it helps to restore independence, dignity and comfort to the many men and women who are affected by these conditions.  To benefit from pelvic muscle retraining, an individual must have some control over their pelvic floor muscles and must be willing to follow a prescribed exercise program.

Pelvic muscle retraining was first used to treat incontinence caused by weak pelvic floor muscles. Weak muscles may lead to accidents or the embarrassing, sometimes noisy loss of gas from the rectum.

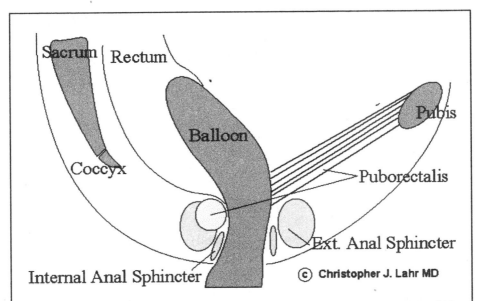

Sacrum | Rectum

Pubis

Balloon

Coccyx

Puborectalis

Ext. Anal Sphincter

Internal Anal Sphincter

© Christopher J. Lahr MD

*Figure 7.1 – Weak Sphincter, Weak Puborectalis During Squeeze.* Side view. Many people (often women) have weak external anal sphincters and weak pelvic diaphragm muscles. These muscles can be weak due to age, inactivity, or birthing injury. When this is the case, even when the person squeezes to try to prevent rectal contents from escaping, the pelvic diaphragm muscles are not strong enough to kink the lower end of the rectum and the external anal sphincter muscle is not strong enough to close the anal canal. These people will suffer from embarrassing incontinence of gas, liquid, or solid rectal contents. Since the pelvic diaphragm muscles and the external anal sphincter muscle are voluntary striated muscles, they can be strengthened by exercise (pelvic muscle retraining) just like the muscles in the arms can be strengthened by doing push-ups and pull-ups. Strengthening the pelvic diaphragm muscles and the external anal sphincter muscle can relieve incontinence. When people are taught to tighten their pelvic diaphragms, however, they must be taught to keep their intra-abdominal muscles relaxed. If they tighten their abdominal wall muscles, then they will increase their intra-abdominal pressure. This will force rectal contents out through the canal with possibly embarrassing results.

#### Chapter 7

If weak muscles are the problem, the goals of pelvic muscle retraining are to:

- strengthen the muscles
- improve the resting tone of the sphincter muscles
- increase the person's ability to contract (squeeze) the muscles
- improve the person's awareness of when it is time to empty the rectum
- decrease the number of accidents.

If constipation or pelvic pain is the problem, the goals of pelvic muscle retraining are to:

- improve the person's awareness of these muscles
- increase a person's ability to keep these muscles in a relaxed position
- promote relaxation when straining to have a bowel movement
- promote more regular bowel movements, and decrease pain or discomfort.

The main focus of pelvic muscle retraining is to teach individuals how to relax and contract (squeeze) the muscles at the anal sphincter. A small sensor is placed at the rectum or vagina. The person stays dressed, and sits in a comfortable lounge chair. The sensor is connected by a cable to a computer. The computer records and measures the muscle movement while the individual watches the computer screen.

When doing these exercises, called Kegel exercises, tighten the pelvic floor muscles as if trying not to pass gas or trying to stop the flow of urine. A woman may feel the muscles tighten around the vagina. A man may feel tightness at the anal sphincter. Try to hold these muscles tight for several seconds while breathing normally and keeping all other muscles relaxed. For example, the abdomen and buttock muscles should stay completely relaxed during this exercise. The only muscle that should feel tight is the muscle at the anal sphincter or the vagina. When the muscles are weak, it is hard to hold them for very long. Gradually, over the course of several weeks (or several months) it is easier to hold the muscles tight for a longer time (up to ten seconds). After tightening the muscles, let go and relax the muscles for ten seconds. If the muscles do not feel completely relaxed after ten seconds, then continue to try to relax them for another ten seconds.

Five repetitions (contract/relax, contract/relax, contract/relax, etc.) make one set of Kegel exercises. Ten sets of Kegel exercises, that is 50 squeezes, should be done each day. A helpful way to remember to do the exercises is to do them once an hour or at various "cues" during the day such as hanging up the phone, stopping at red lights or watching TV commercials. A person can do more sets, up to 100 Kegel exercises daily, as the muscles get stronger. It is important to continue doing these exercises for two to three months to strengthen the pelvic floor muscles adequately. After that time, the exercises must be continued in order to keep the muscles in shape, or they will weaken again. After the symptoms are under control, the exercises should be done at least several days each week.

Some individuals may benefit from using special equipment while doing the exercises at home. However, the average person can do them daily at home without any special equipment.

## Overflow Incontinence

This disorder begins when the person consciously or unconsciously attempts to move their bowels less often. This may be in response to a painful fissure, a painful hemorrhoidectomy wound, or even a painful prostate examination. It can happen in children and in the elderly.

With fewer bowel movements, stool builds up in the rectum. The rectum becomes distended. However, since the distention occurs slowly, the person is not aware of how full the rectum really is.

The large amount of hard stool in the rectum puts pressure on the sphincters, causing leakage. The only time the person recognizes the need to move their bowels is when the sphincter muscles are stretched nearly open. The size and firmness of the stool (impaction) can make removal impossible without medical or manual disimpaction.

Treatment for overflow incontinence starts with manually breaking up the stool. The lower colon is cleaned out with enemas. The person takes stool softeners and fiber. Occasionally, rectal sensation training is necessary to teach the person to recognize smaller rectal volumes.

# 8

# Colon Surgery and Procedures

## Laparoscopy

Colon surgery has been changed by new technology. It can now be done with a laparoscope, a device which has a video camera on its tip. With a laparoscope the surgeon can see inside the abdomen through very small holes in the skin.

Laparoscopy makes surgery easier for the patient. In addition, the surgery that once required a large incision is now done with small surgical instruments through very small incisions that can be covered with adhesive bandages such as Band-Aids and later hidden by a bikini.

## Sigmoidoscopy

Flexible sigmoidoscopy is a procedure using a small, flexible tube with a fiberoptic camera and light attached to its tip to look into the rectum and the colon. The end of the scope can be bent to pass around corners. Flexible sigmoidoscopy is nearly painless, and can be done in the doctor's office.

Using a sigmoidoscope, a doctor can look into the last two feet of the colon for signs of cancer, polyps, diverticulosis or colitis.

The American Cancer Society recommends that from age 40 on, individuals should receive an annual rectal exam. From age 50 on, individuals should have their stool tested for blood annually and should have a flexible sigmoidoscopy every three to five years.

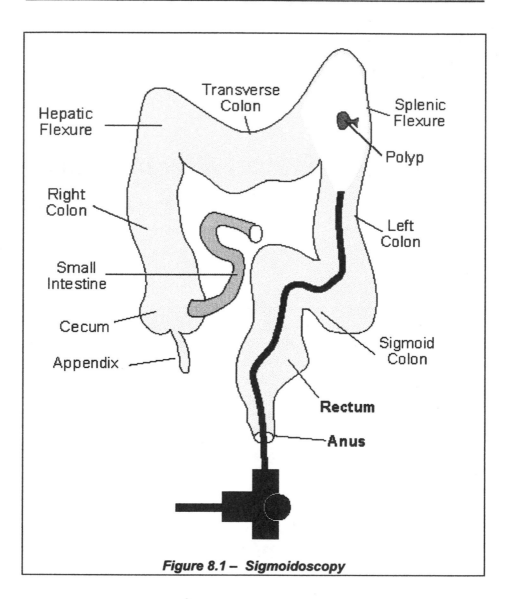

**Figure 8.1 – Sigmoidoscopy**

## Colonoscopy

Colonoscopy is similar to sigmoidoscopy except that it examines the entire colon. Possible reasons for a colonoscopy include rectal bleeding, abdominal pain, diarrhea, and constipation. If these symptoms are minor, do not last long, and go away completely with increased fiber, then colonoscopy may not be necessary. If these symptoms persist, then a colonoscopy may be necessary. Symptoms that can be signs of colon cancer may include rectal bleeding, hidden (occult) blood in the stool, constipation, abdominal pain, change in bowel habits or anemia (low blood count).

Iron deficiency anemia is a sign of blood loss and is also an indication for colonoscopy. Iron deficiency anemia can be caused by bleeding from many sources. Colon and rectal sources of blood lost in the stool include colon and rectal cancer, colon and rectal polyps, inflammatory bowel disease such as ulcerative colitis or Crohn's disease, diverticulosis (sacs in the lining of the colon), hemorrhoids, arteriovenous malformations (small abnormal blood vessels in the lining of the colon), fissure (a crack in the skin at the anal opening), and proctitis (an inflammation of the rectum). Colonoscopy can remove polyps without the need for major surgery.

Colonoscopy is usually done at the hospital as an outpatient procedure, which means that the patient can go home the same day. On the day before the colonoscopy is done, the patient takes a laxative to clean out the colon. In years past, it was necessary to take a gallon of a salty tasting liquid. Now, however, it is necessary to drink only a container of laxative that consists of 2 oz of liquid. For most people, this is much easier to tolerate. Juices and liquids the day before the colonoscopy help to flush the laxative through, and replenish the fluids that the body loses with the laxative.

On the day of the colonoscopy, before the procedure, the patient should not take anything by mouth. This is to avoid getting a sick stomach and vomiting during the procedure. At the hospital, the patient is signed in. Then an IV (intravenous) line (a plastic needle) is placed into the hand or arm. Through this needle we can give medications that cause drowsiness and prevent pain during the procedure.

The patient is brought to the endoscopy room and the physician or nurse gives the medications. The doctor will lubricate the anal canal and pass the colonoscope through the anus into the rectum.

The colonoscope is a long flexible tube with a fiberoptic cord that carries light to the end of it. It also has a computer chip camera on the tip that shows what the inside of the colon looks like. This appears on a computer screen. The colonoscope is controlled by the physician and can be curved to the right, to the left, up or down. The physician steers the scope around corners in the colon.

The colonoscope has a channel (or tunnel) throughout its length, through which tubes, wires and instruments can be passed. This allows the doctor to take biopsies (small pieces of tissue) of anything unusual he might see. This is the way polyps are removed.

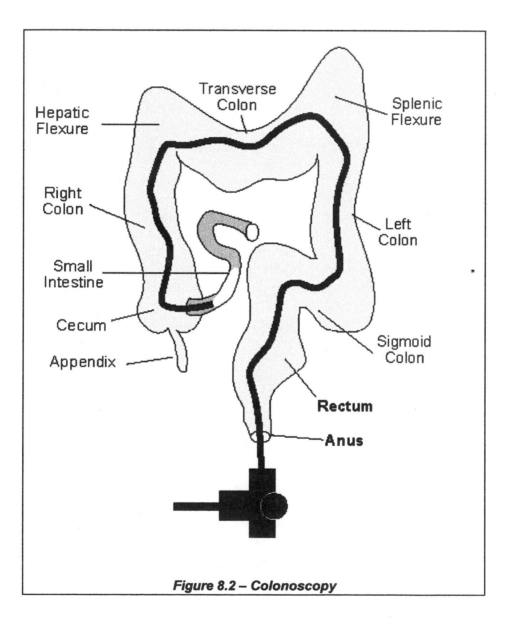

*Figure 8.2 – Colonoscopy*

The colonoscopy usually takes about an hour. After the procedure, the doctor will talk to the patient and a family member. The medicine will prevent the patient from remembering everything the doctor says. There are no restrictions on what can be eaten after the procedure. However, the patient cannot drive the day of the colonoscopy; therefore, he will need a ride home from the hospital.

## Colon Cancer

Colon cancer is a common type of cancer that affects both men and women equally. In 1984, colon cancer and cancer of the rectum were responsible for 14% of cancers in men and 15% of cancers in women. In 1988, there were 147,000 cases of colon cancer, which resulted in 61,500 deaths.

Most colon cancers (93%), occur after age 50; however, it is possible for young people in their 20's to develop colon cancer. The exact causes of colon and rectal cancer are not known. It is believed that certain factors in the diet such as certain chemicals, fats and a low fiber diet cause chromosomal or genetic changes in the cells lining the colon. These changes cause polyps to begin to form. If more genetic changes occur, eventually, cancers will form.

Fiber may cut the risk of colon cancer. In societies such as Japan, where people eat much less meat, milk and fat, the incidence of colon cancer is much lower than it is in the U.S. In countries where people eat large amounts of cereal fiber, the incidence of colon cancer is also much lower.

As is the case with many cancers, the earlier colon cancer is diagnosed, the better the prognosis. The average five-year survival rate of people with colon cancers that are detected early is 75%. If the cancer is not detected early, the average five-year survival rate is 44%.

Colon cancers can be identified at an early stage when they still are very treatable. The smaller a cancer is when it is found, the less likely it is to cause major problems. Stage A colon cancers, which are the smallest and earliest, have not yet invaded the muscle of the colon. People with stage A cancers have an 80% to 90% chance of living five years or longer.

Stage B colon cancers are those which have started to invade the muscle of the colon. People with Stage B have a 60% to 80% chance of living five years or longer.

Stage C cancers of the colon are cancers which have spread to the lymph nodes around the colon. Only 30% to 50% of people with stage C colon cancers will live five years or longer.

## Cancer Risk and Treatment

Colon cancer runs in families. People who have a close relative who has had colon cancer have a 10% risk of developing colon cancer themselves. This means that if you have a mother, father, sister, brother, son or daughter who has had colon cancer, your risk of developing colon cancer is about 10%. However, by being examined frequently and undergoing colonoscopy, you can prevent the development of colon cancer.

Ulcerative colitis is an inflammation of the lining of the colon and if a person has had ulcerative colitis for many years, they have a somewhat higher risk of developing colon cancer.

Screening tests can be done on people who do not have symptoms of cancer. These tests include a stool test, finger rectal examination and proctosigmoidoscopy, or flexible sigmoidoscopy. The Hemoccult test is designed to look for blood hidden in the stool which cannot be seen with the naked eye. Blood can get into the stool either from bleeding in the stomach or bleeding in the intestines. Stomach ulcers can cause blood in the stool as can polyps and cancers in the colon.

A new test is available in which a pellet can be added to the toilet water after the person has a bowel movement. If the water turns blue, this is an indication that there is blood hidden in the stool. If a person does have blood hidden in the stool, it is important to be examined with colonoscopy to look for polyps or cancers.

Radiation therapy is not indicated for most cancers of the colon. In a few cases, when the cancer is in the last six inches of the rectum near the anus and the tumor is very large, radiation therapy, before or after surgery, may be necessary.

Chemotherapy is generally not required for most colon cancers. Recently, however, one specific type of chemotherapy has been shown to improve survival somewhat in persons with stage C cancers of the colon. Stage C cancers are cancers that have spread to the lymph nodes.

Today, very few cancers of the colon require treatment with a permanent colostomy (or permanent bag) unless the cancer is actually growing into the muscles of the anal sphincter. In most cases the cancer can be removed, the colon sewn together again, and the person does not have to have a permanent colostomy.

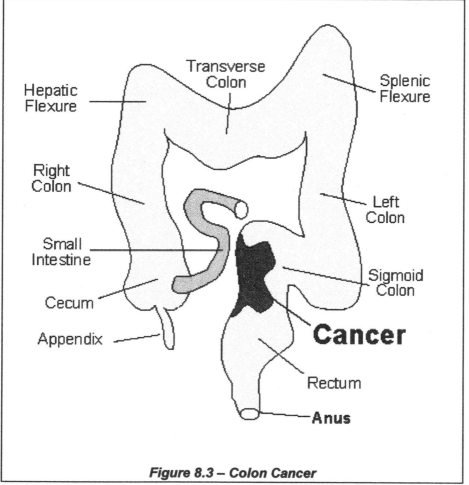

*Figure 8.3 – Colon Cancer*

# Moans, Groans and Stones

In addition to the colon, or large intestine, there are other organs that can cause pain. These can be described by following the path of food and drink through the body, and include the esophagus, the stomach, small intestine, gallbladder, bile ducts, liver, kidneys, urinary bladder, ovaries, uterus and Fallopian tubes.

## Esophagus (Foodpipe)

When you swallow food, it passes down the esophagus or food pipe. The esophagus is a muscular tube that squeezes food down through the chest to the stomach just like a farmer milking a cow. If these muscles do not tighten and relax in a coordinated way, a person will have trouble swallowing.

The esophagus empties into the stomach. At the bottom of the esophagus is a muscle called the lower esophageal sphincter that keeps food from coming back up into the esophagus from the stomach. The stomach is a muscular pouch about the size of a small grocery sack. When it is empty, it does not take up much space; but, it can hold two quarts or more. In the stomach, the food is mixed with acid and enzymes that start to digest the food.

If the lower esophageal sphincter is too weak, then acid from the stomach will be washed up (reflux) into the esophagus. This will cause pain or heartburn. If the muscles of the esophagus are too tight, it may cause chest pain and pain in the upper part of the stomach. This condition can be treated by medicines that relax the muscle.

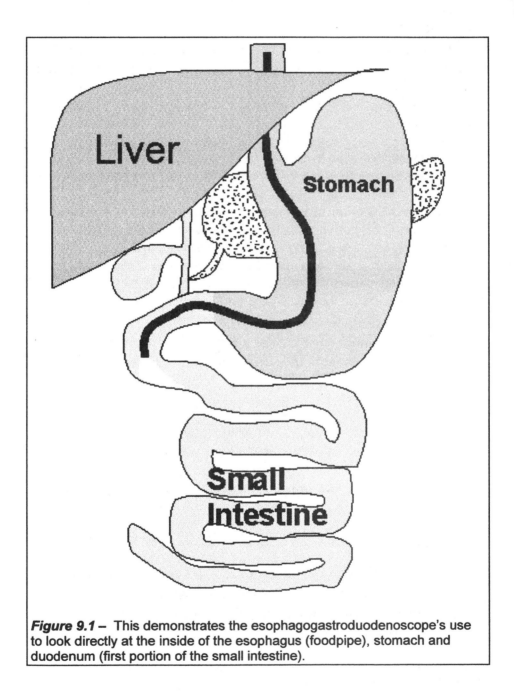

**Figure 9.1 –** This demonstrates the esophagogastroduodenoscope's use to look directly at the inside of the esophagus (foodpipe), stomach and duodenum (first portion of the small intestine).

## *Acid reflux*

The lining of the stomach makes hydrochloric acid to help digest food. Sometimes, the acid in the stomach refluxes into the esophagus. If just a little acid refluxes, the esophagus squeezes it back down. If too much acid refluxes up into the esophagus, it may cause pain or heartburn. Sometimes the acid from the stomach refluxes all the way up into the back of the mouth where you can taste it. This is called water brash. If the acid refluxes into the back of the throat at night it can get into the voice box (larynx) and windpipe (trachea) where it can cause choking or asthma. As many as half of all adult-onset asthma cases are due to reflux. Acid on the vocal cords can cause them to spasm shut causing temporary choking. People who have this condition often have to sleep sitting up in a chair or sitting up in bed.

Acid reflux can also cause burns to the lower part of the esophagus. This can cause it to be red, and can cause ulcers or raw spots in the esophagus. If the problems do not improve with treatment and medication, then a surgical operation, such as a fundoplication, can be performed to prevent acid from washing back up into the esophagus.

Persons with reflux can do several things to reduce the amount of acid in the esophagus:

1) Avoid acid fruit juices such as orange juice or grapefruit juice.

2) Avoid carbonated beverages, such as sodas.

3) Do not eat huge meals that over-fill the stomach.

4) Do not go to bed with a full stomach.

5) Avoid caffeinated beverages, such as coffee.

6) Raise the head of the bed by putting the head of the bed on bricks or cinder blocks.

7) Take prescribed medicines to reduce the acid in the stomach (Prilosec, Pepcid, Prevacid, Tagamet, Zantac, etc.).

8) Take prescribed medicines to strengthen the muscle at the bottom of the esophagus (metaclopramide/Reglan, Propulsid).

9) Take prescribed medicine to help the stomach empty faster (Propulsid, Reglan).

If these measures do not work, and the pain and choking persist, then surgery (fundoplication) may be indicated to relieve the problems.

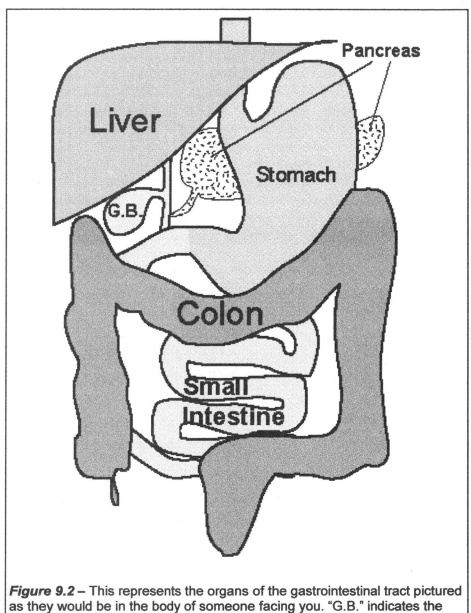

***Figure 9.2*** – This represents the organs of the gastrointestinal tract pictured as they would be in the body of someone facing you. "G.B." indicates the gallbladder.

# Stomach, Gastritis and Ulcers

If the amount of acid in the stomach gets too high, the acid will start to burn a hole in the lining of the stomach. Certain medications such as aspirin, and many medications for arthritis which are called non-steroidal anti-inflammatory agents, weaken the lining of the stomach and make it much more sensitive to acids. Alcohol can also make the stomach lining more sensitive to acids. If the acid in the stomach burns the lining of the stomach for too long, it can result in ulcers which cause pain in the stomach and the back. Eventually, the ulcers can actually perforate or erode a hole in the lining of the stomach.

There is a germ called *Helicobacter pylori* which also makes the lining of the stomach more sensitive to acid. These germs grow in the ulcers in the lining of the stomach and prevent them from healing. Even if the acid in the stomach is reduced, the ulcers generally will not heal as long as the *Helicobacter pylori* germs are present and living in the lining of the stomach.

When there is too much acid in the stomach, and it causes burns or ulcers, the person will notice pain in the upper part of his abdomen just below his rib cage. He may have pain in the left side of his abdomen up under the ribs on the left, or pain in the middle of the back.

Physicians can examine the stomach with a long, flexible narrow tube (scope) that has both a light and a camera at its end. The scope allows us to examine the lining of the stomach for ulcers or inflammation, called gastritis. Gastritis is like a bad sunburn of the skin, except it is on the lining of the stomach and is caused by acid. The lining of the stomach appears red, swollen and irritated.

Small biopsies, which are like tiny bites, are taken from the lining of the stomach. We look at the biopsies under the microscope to see if *Helicobacter pylori* are present.

If *Helicobacter pylori* are present in the lining of the stomach, then in addition to a medication to reduce the amount of acid in the stomach, we also treat the person with other medicines, such as tetracycline, metronidazole and Pepto Bismol, to get rid of the germs.

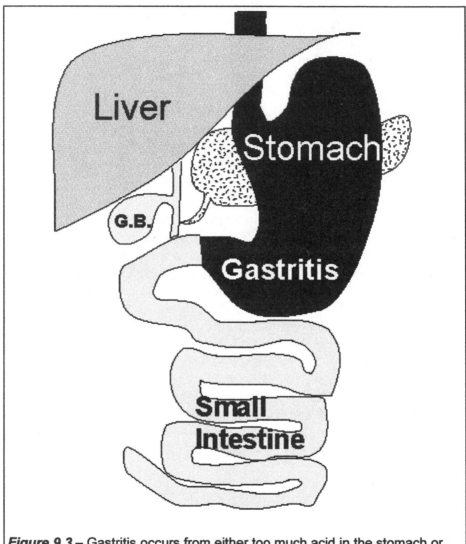

**Figure 9.3** – Gastritis occurs from either too much acid in the stomach or from an infection of the lining of the stomach with a germ called Helicobacter pylori. It is treated with antibiotics if there is H. pylori present. It is always treated with medications which cut down the production of acid by the stomach lining. These medications can include Prevacid, Prilosec, Pepcid, Zantac, Tagamet or Axid.

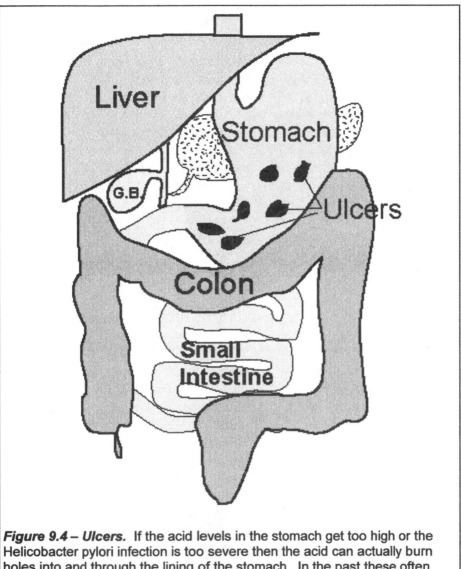

**Figure 9.4 – Ulcers.** If the acid levels in the stomach get too high or the Helicobacter pylori infection is too severe then the acid can actually burn holes into and through the lining of the stomach. In the past these often required surgery. With the modern medications used today to treat gastritis and gastric (stomach) ulcers, surgery can usually be avoided unless the ulcers have burned all the way through the stomach wall.

# Small Intestines

The small intestine connects the stomach to the large intestine (colon). Everything that is useful in the food that we eat is absorbed into the body from the small intestine. Fats, carbohydrates, proteins, and minerals are all absorbed in the body through the lining of the small intestine. Food passes through the small intestine fairly quickly, generally within a few hours of eating. Fortunately, cancer of the small intestine is very unusual.

If a person has had surgery in the abdomen, then scar tissue may form around the small intestine, causing it to become kinked or blocked. This is called a small bowel obstruction and can cause crampy pain. If the small intestine is completely blocked, surgery is required to remove the scar tissue.

# Gallbladder, Bile Ducts and Liver

Another cause of pain in the upper abdomen, especially in the right side on the ribs, is gallbladder disease. The liver is located up under the ribs on the right side of the abdomen, and makes chemicals which help to digest food in the intestines. The liver is connected to the first part of the small intestine, called the duodenum, by a tube called the common bile duct. Bile made in the liver passes through the common bile duct into the small intestine.

Protected on one side of the common bile duct is a small pouch one to three inches in length, called the gallbladder. Between meals, a small valve at the end of the common bile duct closes, and the bile goes into the gallbladder. In the gallbladder, the bile is concentrated (thickened) and stored until the next meal. When food from the stomach enters the duodenum, the gallbladder squeezes out the bile through the common bile duct into the duodenum where it helps in the digestion of food.

The bile contains salts, fats and cholesterol. Sometimes, the concentration or mixture of these various chemicals changes which allows little crystals to form in the bile. These crystals grow to form small rocks or "stones." These stones can be very small, as small as a grain of sand, or they can be as large as golf balls. If these stones get caught in the opening of the gallbladder when the gallbladder squeezes, then the gallbladder cannot empty, and this causes severe pain. Sometimes, the stones are caught in the common bile duct. This causes bile to build up in the liver.

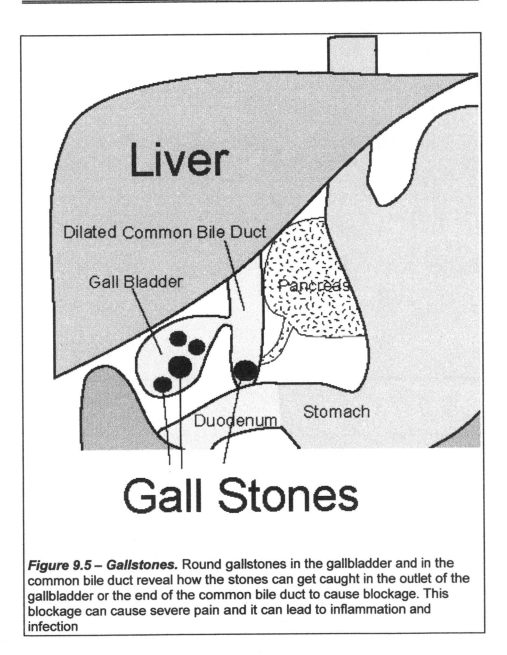

**Gall Stones**

*Figure 9.5 – Gallstones.* Round gallstones in the gallbladder and in the common bile duct reveal how the stones can get caught in the outlet of the gallbladder or the end of the common bile duct to cause blockage. This blockage can cause severe pain and it can lead to inflammation and infection

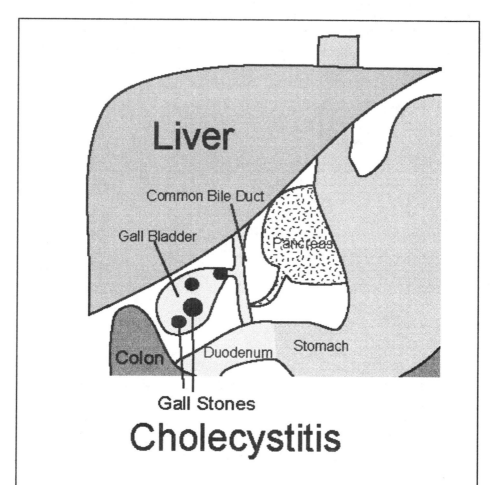

Liver

Common Bile Duct

Gall Bladder

Pancreas

Colon

Duodenum

Stomach

Gall Stones

# Cholecystitis

**Figure 9.6 – Bile Build-Up.** The stones in the gallbladder and in the common bile duct have caused obstruction of these two structures causing bile to build up under pressure. This pressure can cause pain. Since the bile just sits there without the normal emptying flow it can become infected by germs. This infection can spread to the liver (ascending cholangitis) and cause life-threatening problems.

When stones are present in the gallbladder and they are causing pain, they should be removed. Just a few years ago, it required major surgery with a long painful incision in the upper abdomen to remove the gallbladder and the gallstones. With the invention of laparoscopic cholecystectomy, however, we can now remove the gallbladder through small puncture holes, and a big incision is not necessary.

If there are stones in the common bile duct, a gastroenterologist can look down into the small intestine and into the common bile duct with a scope, and the stones can be removed by widening the opening of the common bile duct at the duodenum. The person can usually go home the day following this procedure.

## Kidneys

Another cause of abdominal pain may be problems with the kidneys. The kidneys are two bean-shaped organs that sit in the middle of the back, one on each side of the backbone. They filter the blood and remove wastes from it. They are about four to six inches in length and are connected by two tubes (ureters) to the bladder. If stones are formed by crystals in the urine, they can get caught in the ureter and can cause severe pain. This pain is generally felt in the middle of the back. It can also be felt in the lower abdomen and the groins.

## Urinary Bladder

The urinary bladder is located in the middle of the pelvis. It is in front of the vagina and uterus in a woman, and in front of the rectum in a man. This organ holds the body's urine. If the bladder or urine becomes infected, the result could be a burning sensation and pain. This condition can also cause bleeding. The bladder can be examined with an instrument called a cystoscope, and polyps or cancers can be identified and removed.

## Ovaries, Uterus and Fallopian Tubes

The uterus is located in the mid-pelvis just behind the bladder. This is the muscular cavity in which a fetus (baby) grows and lives until it is born. The muscle in the uterus can grow abnormally to cause fibroids which may cause pain and swelling.

The ovaries produce eggs from which babies are born. Every month while a woman is menstruating, small cysts form on the ovaries. These cysts release the eggs. Sometimes these cysts, which are just small sacs of fluid, can get large and become painful.

The eggs which come from the ovaries get to the uterus through the Fallopian tubes. These are small tubes and can get infected and cause inflammation and pain in the pelvis. If the fertilized egg gets stuck in the Fallopian tube instead of passing all the way to the uterus, then the embryo can start to grow in the Fallopian tube. This can cause serious trouble such as bleeding and pain. This condition must be treated surgically.

## Colon-Rectal Surgeon

The colon-rectal surgeon has had specialized training specifically in problems of the colon, rectum and anus. He sees problems every day with which others are not familiar. Because he is a surgeon, he can both identify the problems and do the surgery to correct them. In addition, since he knows the most effective treatments currently available, he is better able to help people avoid surgery whenever possible.

## Medications that Alter Bowel Function

Medicines that alter bowel function can be divided into two groups. Laxatives are medications that speed up the bowels, and anti-diarrheals are medications that slow the bowels. The following partial list gives an idea of medications available.

### Laxatives

*Psyllium* is a fiber supplement and stool normalizer. It prevents stools from being too soft or too hard. Sometimes psyllium and other fiber products may actually make the constipation worse. If psyllium makes constipation worse, then one should see a physician.

*Lactulose* is a sugar syrup not absorbed into the body. It passes into the colon where it pulls water from the intestinal lining into the stool. This makes the stool softer and more liquid.

*Mineral oil* is an oil not absorbed into the body. In the colon, it acts as a lubricant.

*Stimulant laxatives* include substances such as senna, herbal teas and over-the-counter laxatives, Ex-Lax, Correctol and Dulcolax. They cause the colon to pump harder and faster. Frequent regular use of these medications over a long period of time may cause the colon to become unresponsive to them.

*Golytely and Colyte* are laxatives used to clean out the colon prior to colonoscopy, barium enema or surgery. They are powders mixed with water. Chemicals in the powder prevent the water from being absorbed into the body. Therefore, it stays inside the colon and washes out the stool. They come in several flavors. They can be used on a regular basis to help relieve constipation.

Some medications seem to effect the muscles of the stomach and intestines. These include erythromycin, Cytotec, Reglan and Propulsid. Unfortunately, their effect upon constipation has not been consistent.

### Anti-Diarrheals

*Psyllium* is a fiber supplement and a stool normalizer and is one of the most effective agents to treat diarrhea. *Lomotil* and *Imodium* are non-narcotics that slow movement in the intestines.

*Paregoric* and codeine are narcotics that slow the movement in the bowels. *Codeine* (30 mg), when used with salt tablets (500 mg), four times a day can also be very effective.

*Questran* is an agent that binds to bile salts in the intestines and prevents these bile salts from stimulating the colon. *Carafate* protects bowel surfaces and sometimes relieves diarrhea.

## Pancreatitis

At the Medical University of South Carolina (MUSC), where I am on staff, we have recently been doing a diagnostic procedure called *endoscopic ultrasound*. In this procedure a special endoscope with an ultrasound probe on the end is passed into the stomach. The stomach is right next to the pancreas in the abdominal cavity. Therefore, the ultrasound probe on end of the scope can be placed right against the pancreas. This allows then to take very accurate pictures of the pancreas. This has allowed us to see problems in the pancreas that could not be seen before.

We have found that many patients who have slow colons and severe abdominal pain also have problems with their pancreas called *chronic pancreatitis*. This is a pancreatitis that is **not** caused by alcohol or by gallstones.

The pancreas makes insulin and it also makes enzymes to help digest food. Lipase is an enzyme that digests fat. Amylase is an enzyme that digests carbohydrates. These enzymes are produced by the pancreas. They can be measured in the blood. Sometimes when the pancreas is suddenly injured the levels of amylase and lipase in the blood will be markedly elevated.

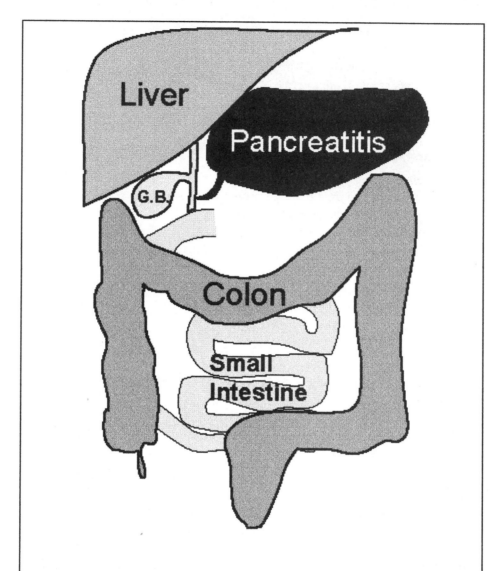

***Figure 9.7 – Pancreatitis.*** If the opening of the pancreas duct (which drains the enzymes the pancreas makes) becomes blocked, it could lead to very painful inflammation or irritation. The pancreas duct can be blocked by gallstones or the muscle that closes the duct can become too tight and this can block the duct. Alcohol can also irritate the pancreas, causing pancreatitis.

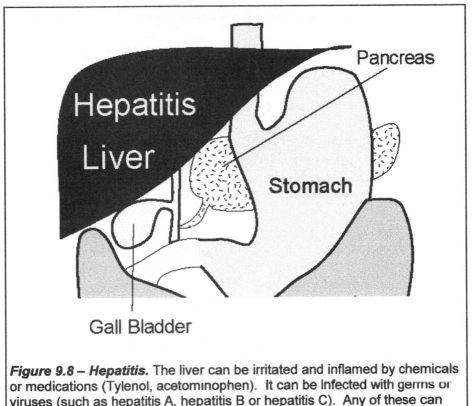

*Figure 9.8 – Hepatitis.* The liver can be irritated and inflamed by chemicals or medications (Tylenol, acetominophen). It can be infected with germs or viruses (such as hepatitis A, hepatitis B or hepatitis C). Any of these can cause hepatitis with severe weakness, fatigue, nausea and sometimes pain.

The pancreas makes the enzymes then the enzymes are collected in a small tube called the pancreatic duct. This duct carries the enzymes to the first part of the small intestine called the duodenum. Here the enzymes are activated and they digest foods in the intestine. If the end of the duct is blocked then the enzymes get trapped in the pancreas. They can become activated and digest the pancreas itself causing pancreatitis and severe pain.

At the end of the pancreatic duct just as it enters the duodenum there is a ring of muscle around the duct. This is a sphincter muscle. It is called a sphincter muscle because when it contracts, it squeezes the end of the duct closed. The anal sphincter acts in a similar way to close the rectum. The pancreatic duct sphincter opens up when someone eats food so that the pancreatic enzymes can leave the pancreas and get to the food. If the pancreatic duct sphincter doesn't open then problems may occur when the enzymes can't get out.

If the pancreas is injured by gallstones blocking the pancreatic duct or by alcohol or by narrowing of the end of the pancreatic duct then the enzymes for digesting food can be activated and can start to digest the pancreas. This causes severe pain in the pancreas which is felt in the upper abdomen and through to the back.

In years past the only way we had to measure injury or inflammation to the pancreas was by measuring elevated levels of amylase and lipase in the blood. Sometimes if the pancreas was very, very swollen or if the pancreas had been inflamed a long time then calcium buildup would be present that could be seen on CAT scan. Many patients, however, had pain in the upper part of the abdomen that got worse with eating and went through to their back. This sounded like pancreatitis but amylase levels, lipase levels and CAT scans were normal because these tests were not very sensitive.

With the *endoscopic ultrasound* (EUS) expert pancreatic doctors discovered that they could see pancreatitis present in some patients even when blood amylase levels, blood lipase levels and pancreatic CAT scans were normal. Many patients had had pain for some time that no one could figure out. When EUS was done and pancreatitis was found the pain was explained.

Discovering the pancreatitis is important because it can be treated. If pancreatitis is present then doctors can do an ERCP (endoscopic retrograde cholangiopancreatogram) to look at the duct of the pancreas. In this procedure an endoscope is passed through the mouth, throat and stomach into the duodenum. Here a small tube is placed into the pancreatic duct and the biliary duct (which goes to the liver). X-ray dye is injected through this tube into the ducts so that they can be seen on an x-ray screen. If the duct is blocked by a stone the stone can be removed with special instruments and the scope. If the duct is blocked by scar tissue, or by a pancreatic sphincter that is too tight, then the pancreatic sphincter can be opened with a small electrical knife through the ERCP scope.

Opening a closed pancreatic sphincter will allow the pancreatic enzymes to leave the pancreas as they should and enter the duodenum to digest food. If a patient has been suffering from pancreatitis due to a blocked pancreatic duct then unblocking the duct will stop the injury to the duct and allow it to begin healing. It may take several weeks or more sometimes for the inflammation and swelling to resolve. It is just like a twisted sprained ankle. After it is once sprained even though you may not twist it any more it still takes a while for the swelling to go down and for the pain to go away.

There are other medications that we use to treat pancreatitis. These medications include pancreozymin, amitriptylline and somatostatin. Pancreozymin contains multiple enzymes like lipase and others that help digest food. In this way the pancreas doesn't have to make as many enzymes. This lets the pancreas rest and heal.

Somatostatin is a natural body hormone that turns the pancreas off. It must be given with a needle into the skin two or three times a day.

Amitriptylline is a medicine originally used as an antidepressant that also appears to have an effect on relieving pancreatic pain.

Resting the pancreas allows it to heal. One thing that allows the pancreas to rest is avoiding any food by mouth. Obviously a person would starve if this went on for long. Therefore one of the measures we take in bad cases of pancreatitis is to give all of a person's nutrition by vein. This is called hyperalimentation. This must be done through a vein in the chest under the collarbone. Doctors can place a small implantable port just under the skin in the chest. When a person needs his nutrition a short small needle is passed through the skin into the port. The port is connected by a small catheter (tube) to a vein in the chest. The hyperalimentation is given through the needle into the port through the catheter into the vein. This allows a person to eat little or nothing and still stay healthy and maintain their weight. This can be done at home during the night. The person can then go out and function during the day because the needle is removed from the port and they are not connected to anything.

One important factor in allowing the pancreas to heal is avoiding things that irritate it or stimulate it. Alcohol strongly irritates the pancreas. Fatty foods stimulate the pancreas to produce enzymes. Many patients describe severe pain coming on 10-30 minutes after eating.

Once the inflammation of pancreatitis resolves then usually the patient can return to a usual diet. This may take several months though.

We have seen that a percentage of patients with colonic inertia (slow colon) have been found to have chronic pancreatitis. Some of them have had severe attacks of pain that have lasted many weeks. In years past when we saw these patients with pain none of the tests showed anything abnormal because the only tests available for the pancreas were CAT scans, amylase levels and lipase levels. These would all be normal. Now that we have

EUS available we are able to identify the patients with pancreatitis. Once we know pancreatitis is present we can treat it with ERCP, sphincterotomy and medications.

The pain from pancreatitis can be so severe that often strong pain medications are required. Sometimes persons must be hospitalized for intravenous pain medications.

## A Long, Happy Life

When one considers the advancements in medical technology of today, the expertise of a competent colon-rectal surgeon, the benefits of having regular check ups, and the availability of educational material concerning colon-rectal problems, it is possible for you and your loved ones to better manage colon and rectal problems and live longer, happier lives.

# References

**RECTOPEXY AND SIGMOIDECTOMY FOR DIFFICULT RECTAL EMPTYING**

1. Drossman DA, Li Z, Andruzzi E, Temple RD, Talley NJ, Thompson WG, Whitehead WE, Janssens J, Funch-Jensen P, Corazziari E, Richter JE and Koch GG. U.S. household survey of functional gastrointestinal disorders. Prevalence, Sociodemography and Health Impact. Dig Dis Sci 1993; 38(9): 1569-80.

2. Enck P. Biofeedback Training in Disordered Defecation: A Critical Review. Dig Dis Sci 1993;38:1953-1960.

3. Goldberg SM, Gordon PH, Nivatvongs S. Rectal Prolapse. Essentials of anorectal surgery. J.B. Lippincott Company. Philadelphia and Toronto. 248-268. 1980.

4. Fleshman JW, Fry RD, Kodner IJ. The Surgical Management of Constipation. Bailliere's Clinical Gastroenterology 1992;6(1):145-162.

5. Orrom WJ, Bartolo DCC, Miller R, Mortensen, Roe AM. Rectopexy Is an Ineffective Treatment for Obstructed Defecation. Dis Col Rec 1991;34: 41-46.

6. Heine JA, Wong WD, Goldberg SM. Surgical Treatment for Constipation. Surg, Gyn Ob 1993;176:403-410.

7. Frykman, HM, Abdominal proctopexy and primary sigmoid resection for rectal procidentia. Am J Surg1955;90:780.

8. Frykman HM, Goldberg SM. The surgical treatment of rectal procidentia. Surg Gynecol Obstet 1969;129:1225.

9. Goldberg SM, Gordon PH. Treatment of rectal prolapse. Clin Gastroenterol 1975;4:489.

10. Madoff RD, Williams JG, Wong WD, Rothenberger DA, Goldberg SM. Long-Term Functional Results of Colon Resection and Rectopexy for Overt Rectal Prolapse. Am J Gastro 1992;87(1):101-104.

11. Huber FT, Stein H, Siewert JR. Functional Results after Treatment of Rectal Prolapse with Rectopexy and Sigmoid Resection. World J Surg 1995;19:138-143.

## The History of Rectal Suspension for Rectal Descent

Ball, Charles, The Rectum, 1910.

Findlay, Leonard. Lancet, 1923, **1**, 76; the Clinical Study and Treatment of Sick Children, p. 141 (Oliver & Boyd, Edinburgh, 1934)

Frykman, HM, Abdominal proctopexy and primary sigmoid resection for rectal procidentia. Am J Surg1955;90:780.

Frykman HM, Goldberg SM. The surgical treatment of rectal procidentia. Surg Gynecol Obstet 1969;129:1225.

Gabriel William B. The Principles and Practice of Rectal Surgery. 1948. Charles C. Thomas. Springfield, Illinois, USA.

Goldberg SM, Gordon PH. Treatment of rectal prolapse. Clin Gastroenterol 1975;4:489.

Graham, Roscoe R. Ann. of Surg., 1942, 115, 1007.

Hartmann, Chirurgie du Rectum, 1931, p. 147.

Hoffman MJ, Kodner IJ, Fry RD. Internal intussusception of the rectum: diagnosis and surgical management. Dis Colon Rectum 1984; **27**:435-441.

Ihre T. Internal procidentia of the rectum-treatment and results. Scand J Gastroenterol 7: 643, 1972.

Ihre T, Seligson U. Intussusception of the rectum-internal procidentia: treatment and results in 90 patients. Dis Colon Rectum 1975, **18**, 391-396.

Moschcowitz, Alexis V. Surg. Gyn. and Obst., 1912, **15**, 7.

Nichols, R.J., Simson, J.N.L. Anteroposterior rectopexy in the treatment of solitary rectal ulcer syndrome without overt rectal prolapse. Br. J. Surg. 1986, **73**, 222-224.

Quénu, E. Révue de Chirurgie, 1882,2, 173.

Pemberton, J. de J., and Stalker, L.K. Ann. of Surg., 1939, **109**, 799.

Madoff RD, Williams JG, Wong WD, Rothenberger DA, Goldberg SM. Long-Term Functional Results of Colon Resection and Rectopexy for Overt Rectal Prolapse. Am J Gastro 1992;87(1):101-104.

Ripstein CB. Treatment of massive rectal prolapse. Am J Surg. 83: 68, 1952.

## TOTAL COLECTOMY FOR COLONIC INERTIA

1. Wexner SD, Daniel N, Jagelman DG. Colectomy for constipation: physiologic investigation is the key to success. Dis Colon Rectum 1991;34:851-856.

2. Kamm MA, Hawley PR, Lennard-Jones JE. Outcome of colectomy for severe idiopathic constipation. Gut 1988; 29:969-973.

3. Howard RJ, Davis RH, Clench MH, Mathias JR. Subtotal colectomy as a therapeutic consideration in patients with chronic obstipation refractory to medical therapy. Gastroenterology, 1985, 88:1423.

4. Schuffler MD, Krishnamurthy S. Constipation and colectomy. Dig Dis Sci 1988; 33:1197-1198.

5. Metcalf AM, Phillips SF, Zinsmeister AR, MacCarty RL, Beart RW, Wolff BG. Simplified assessment of segmental colonic transit. Gastroenterology 1987;92:40-47.

6. Camilleri M, Thompson WG, Fleshman JW, Pemberton JH. Clinical management of intractable constipation. Ann Intern Med. 1994; 121:520-528.

7. Talley NJ, Weaver AL, Zinmeister AR, Melton LJ 3d. Functional constipation and outlet delay: a population based study. Gastroenterology. 1993; 105;781-90.

8. Drossman DA, Zhiming LI, Andruzzi E, Temple RD, Talley NJ, Thompson WG, Whitehead WE, Janssens J, Funch-Jensen P, Corazziari E, Richter JE, Koch GG. U.S. householder survey of functional gastrointestinal disorders. Prevalence, sociodemography, and health impact. Dig Dis Sci. 1993;38:1569-80.

9. Thompson WG, Heaton KW. Functional bowel disorders in apparently healthy people. Gastroenterology 1980;79:283-288.

10. Murtagh J. Constipation. Australian Fam Physician 1990; 19:1693-7.

11. Bleijenberg G, Kuijpers HC. Treatment of spastic pelvic floor syndrome with biofeedback. Dis Col Rectum 1987;30:108-111.

12. Preston DM, Hawley PR, Lennard-Jones JE, Todd IP. Results of colectomy for severe idiopathic constipation in women (Arbuthnot Lane's disease). Br J Surg 1984; 71:547-552.

13. Beck DE, Jagelman DG, Fazio VW. The surgery of idiopathic constipation. Gastroenterol Clin North Am 1987; 16:143-156.

14. Leon SH, Krishnamurthy S, Schuffler MD. Subtotal colectomy for severe idiopathic constipation: a followup study of 13 patients. Dig Dis Sci 1987;32: 1249-1254.

15. Vasilevsky CA, Nemer FD, Balcos EG, Christenson CD, Goldberg SM. Is subtotal colectomy a viable option in the management of chronic constipation? Dis Colon Rectum 1988;31:679-681.

16. Akerval S, Fasth S, Nordren S, and others. The functional results after colectomy and ileorectal anastomosis for severe constipation (Arbuthot Lane's disease) as related to rectal sensory function. Int J Colorect Dis 1988;3:96-101.

17. Yoshioka K, Keighley MRB. Clinical results of colectomy for severe constipation. Br J Surg 1989;76:600-604.

18. Heine JA, Wong WD, Goldberg SM. Surgical treatment for constipation. Surgery, Gynecology and Obstetrics 1993;176:403-410.

19. Lane RHS, Todd IP. Idiopathic megacolon: a review of 42 cases. Br J Surg 1977; 64:305-310.

20. McCready RA, Beart RW. The surgical treatment of incapacitating constipation associated with idiopathic megacolon. Mayo Clin Proc 1979; 54:779-783.

21. Arbuthnot Lane W. Results of the operative treatment of chronic constipation. Br Med J 1908;1:126-130.

## REFERENCES: PELVIC MUSCLE RETRAINING

Wexner SD, Daniel N, Jagelman DG. Colectomy for constipation: physiologic investigation is the key to success. Dis Colon Rectum 1991;34:851-856.

Wald A, Caruana BJ, Reimanis MG, Bauman DH and Hinds JP. Contributions of evacuation proctography and anorectal manometry to evaluation of adults with constipaation and defecatory difficulty. Dig Dis Sci, 1990; 35:481-487.

Wald A. Colonic transit and anorectal manometry in chronic idiopathic constipation. Arch Intern Med, 1986, 146: 1713-1716.

Bleijenberg G, Kuijpers HC. Treatment of spastic pelvic floor syndrome with biofeedback. Dis Colon Rectum 1987;30:108-11.

Roberts PL, Coller JA, Schoetz DJ, Veidenheimer MC. Manometric assessment of paatients with obstetric injuries and fecal incontinence. Dis Colon Rectum 1990;33:16-20.

Williams JG, Wong WD, Jensen L, Rothenberger DA, Goldberg SM: Incontinence and rectal prolapse: a prospective manometric sstudy. Dis Colon Rectum 1991;34:209-216.

Whitehead WE, Burgio KI, Engel BT: Biofeedback treatment of fecal incontinence in geriatric patients. J Am Ger Soc 1985;33:3204.

Loening-Bauke V: Efficacy of biofeedback training in improving fecal incontinence and anorectal physiologic function. Gut 1990;31:1395-1402.

Loening-Bauke V: Biofeedback therapy for fecal incontinece. Dig Dis 1990; 7:112-24.

Kegel AH: Progressive exercise in the functional restoration of the perineal muscle. Am J Ob Gyn 1948; 56:238-48.

Macleod JH: Management of anal incontinence by biofeedback. Gastroenterology 1987; 93:291-4.

Miner PB, Donnelly TC, Read NW: Investigation of mode of action of biofeedback in treatment of fecal incontinence. Dig Dis Sci 1990; 35(10):1291-98.

Prospective study of conservative and operative treatment for fecal incontinence. British J Surgery. 1988; 75:101-5.

Tries J: Kegel exercises enhanced by biofeedback. J Enterostom Ther 1990;17:67-76.

McHugh S, Kersey K, Diamant NE: Biofeedback training for fecal incontinence. Outcome according to physiological parameters. Gastroenterology 1988;94:4295.

Kuijpers HC. Application of colorectal laboratory in diagnosis aand treatment of functional constipation. Dis Colon Rectum 1990; 33:35-9.

Cerulli MA, Nikoomanesh P, Schuster MM. Progress in biofeedback conditioning for fecal incontinence. Gastroenterol 1979; 76:742-6.

Engel BT, Nikoomanesh P, Schuster MM. Operant condition of rectosphincteric responses in the treatment of fecal incontinence. New Engl J Med 1974; 290:646-9.

Weber J, Ducrotte PH, Touchais JY, Roussignol C, Denis PH. Biofeedback training for constipation in adults and children. Dis Colon Rectum 1987; 30: 844-6.

Heyman S, Wexner S. EMG training for paradoxical puborectalis in patients with chronic constipation. Biof Self-Regulation 1990; 15:64-5.

Leoning-Baucke V. Modulation of abnormal defecation dynamics by biofeedbaack treatment in chronically constipated children with encopresis. J Pediatr 1990; 116:214-22.

Wexner SD, et al . A prospective assessment of biofeedback for the treatment of paradoxical puborectalis contraction. Dis Colon Rectum 1992; 35(2):145-50.

Ger GC, et al. Evaluation and treatment of chronic intractable rectal pain. Dis Colon Rectum 1993; 36(2)

Jorge JMN et al. Fecal incontinence: current status. Dis Colon Rectum 1993; 36(1) 77-79.

Ger GC, et al. Anorectal manometry in the diagnosis of paradoxical puborectalis syndrome. Dis Colon Rectum 1993; 36(2): 139-45.

Wexner SD, Daniel N, Jagelman DG. Colectomy for constipation: physiologic investigation is the key to success. Dis Colon Rectum 1991;34:851-856.

Vasilevsky CA, Nemer FD, Balcos EG, Christenson CD, Goldberg SM. Is subtotal colectomy a viable option in the management of chronic constipation? Dis Colon Rectum 1988;31:679-681.

Kamm MA, Hawley PR, Lennard-Jones JE. Outcome of colectomy for severe idiopathic constipation. Gut 1988; 29:969-973.

Heine JA, Wong WD, Goldberg SM. Surgical treatment for constipation. Gynecology and Obstetrics 1993;176:403-410.

Leon SH, Krishnamurthy S, Schuffler MD. Subtotal colectomy for severe idiopathic constipation: a followup study of 13 patients. Dig Dis Sci 1987;32: 1249-1254.

Preston DM, Hawley PR, Lennard-Jones JE, Todd IP. Results of colectomy for severe idiopathic constipation in women (Arbuthnot Lane's disease). Br J Surg 1984; 71:547-552.

Preston DM , Lennard-Jones JE. Severe chronic constipation of young women: 'idiopathic slow transit constipation.' Gut 1986, 27: 41-48.

McCready RA, Beart RW. The surgical treatment of incapacitating constipation associated with idiopathic megacolon. Mayo Clin Proc 1979; 54:779-783.

Lane RHS, Todd IP. Idiopathic megacolon: a review of 42 cases. Br J Surg 1977; 64:305-310.

a.  Sonnenberg A, Koch TR.  Epidemiology of constipation in the United States. Dis Colon Rectum 1989;32:1-8.

b.  Lahr CJ, Rothenberger DA, Jensen LL, Goldberg SM.  Balloon topography: a simple method of evaluating anal function.  Dis Colon Rectum 1986;29:1-5.

c.  Lahr CJ, Cherry DA, Jensen LL, Rothenberger DA.  Balloon sphincterography: clinical findings after 200 patients.  Dis Colon Rectum 1988; 31:347-351.

d.  Bleijenberg G, Kuijpers JH.  Treatment of the spastic pelvic floor syndrome using biofeedback.  Ned Tijdschr Geneeskd.  1987;131:446-9.

e.  Bleijenberg G, Kuijpers HC.  Treatment of the spastic pelvic floor syndrome with biofeedback.  Dis Col Rect.  1987;30:108-111.

f.  Vesilevsky CA, Nemer FD, Balcos EG, Christenson CE, Goldberg SM.  Is subtotal colectomy a viable option in the management of chronic constipation? Dis Col Rect.  1988;31:679-681.

g.  MacLeod JH.  Management of anal incontinence by biofeedback. Gastroenterology 1987;93:291-4.

h.  Whitehead WE, Burgio KL, Engel BT.  Biofeedback treatment of fecal incontinence in geriatric patients.  J Am Geriatr Soc 1985; 33:320-4.

i.  Wald A, Tunuguntla, AK.  Anorectal sensorimotor dysfunction in fecal incontinence and diabetes mellitus.  N Engl J Med 1984; 310:1282-7.

j.  Buser WD, Miner PB.  Delayed rectal sensation with fecal incontinence. Gastroenterology 1986;91:1186-1191.

k.  Snooks SJ, Swash M, Setchell M, Henry MM.  Injury to innervation of pelvic floor sphincter musculature in childbirth.  Lancet 1984; ii:546-550.  8 September.

# Glossary

**Abscess** – Collection of pus in the flesh. Must be treated with surgery to let out the pus.

**Anal crypt** – small oil glands in the skin of the opening of the anal canal. If germs are forced into the crypts by hard bowel movements then the germs can fester causing fistulas and abscesses.

**Anal electromyography** – Measurement of the electrical activity of the anal sphincter muscles. This test is very useful in making sure that the sphincter muscles relax like they should during bowel movements.

**Anal manometry** – Non-X-ray measurement of the anal canal pressures. Both internal and external anal sphincter strength is measured.

**Anal papilla** – Small finger-like projections into the anal canal normally present. If they become inflamed or enlarged and tender they can be painful and require removal. These are called hypertrophied anal papilla.

**Anal stenosis** – Narrowing of the anal opening causing difficult rectal emptying.

**Anoscopy** – Office diagnostic procedure in which a short two and one half inch scope is placed inside the anal canal to examine the anal canal and determine the size of internal hemorrhoids.

**Barium enema** – X-ray of the colon in which liquid that shows up on X-rays is inserted into the colon. This gives a shadow picture of the colon. Colon tumors and large polyps can be seen with this technique. Sometimes deep ulcers and changes in the lining of the colon can also be seen with this technique.

**Cecum** – The very first part of the colon. The small intestine pumps its contents into the cecum. The cecum is the widest portion of the colon.

**Cecal bascule** – Abnormal excess mobility of the cecum caused by inadequate attachments of the cecum to the body wall. This results in a cecum that can swing around the abdominal cavity and in doing so can kink the colon farther down the line at the point around which the cecum is swinging.

**Coccygodynia** – Pain in the tailbone (coccyx) due to injury or inflammation of the coccyx and the joint between the coccyx and the sacrum. It can be treated by anti-inflammatory medications, injection of the joint and coccyx with steroids or with surgical removal of the coccyx.

**Colonic inertia** – Slow colon that causes severe constipation due to very infrequent bowel movements. the colon does not pump its contents through with the speed it should to prevent constipation.

**Colonoscopy** – Outpatient diagnostic procedure in which a fiberoptic light and camera in a long flexible tube is inserted through the colon while the patient sleeps. This allows the doctor to see the entire lining of the colon and remove small and medium sized polyps through the scope without the need for surgery. Cancer, polyps, diverticulosis and colitis can be seen in this manner. Biopsies can be performed.

**Crohn's Disease** – Inflammation of the intestines (colon or small intestine) with no known cause which can result in abdominal pain, rectal bleeding, diarrhea or anal fistulas.

**Defecography** – X-ray diagnostic procedure in which paste that shows up on X-rays is placed into the rectum, the vagina, the sigmoid colon, the bladder and the small intestine. The person then expels the paste in the rectum while sitting on a specially designed toilet seat while video X-rays are taken. These video X-rays show the shape of the rectum as it empties. Rectoceles, enteroceles, sigmoidoceles, rectal descent and intussusception can be seen with defecography. Defecography is the single most important test for evaluating difficult rectal emptying.

**Dentate line** – Dividing line between the anal skin and the rectal lining. The dentate line is where anal crypts and anal papillae are located. It is here that most fistulas start out.

**Diverticulitis** – Inflammation and infection of diverticulosis that can cause pain and tenderness. It can lead to abscess formation or perforation of the colon requiring surgery.

**Diverticulosis** – Small sacs through the wall of the colon caused by high pressures inside the colon from not enough fiber in the diet.

**Enterocele** – Bulging of the small intestines into weak spots in the pelvic floor caused by inadequate support of the rectum, vagina and urinary bladder. If it is causing symptoms then it can be treated by resuspending the pelvic organs from the bones of the pelvis.

**External anal sphincter muscle** – Voluntary muscle that keeps the anal opening closed during heavy lifting, straining, coughing or vigorous activity. It also is the muscle contracted when the rectum is full and a person is rushing to get to the bathroom in time.

**External hemorrhoids** – Swollen anal skin that may become irritated and tender.

**Feces** (pronounced *fee-sees*) – Waste material excreted from the bowel.

**Fecal incontinence** – Involuntary and unwanted expulsion or leakage of rectal contents. It can be caused by weakness of the anal sphincter muscles but may also be due to rectal problems which cause stool to back up in the rectum because the rectum won't properly empty.

**Fissure** – Crack in the anal skin caused by bowel movements that are too hard or too liquid.

**Fistula** – Infected tunnel through the flesh and skin in the anal area. These occur when germs in hard bowel movements get driven into glands inside the anal opening then the germs fester and work their way out to the anal skin. Fistulas can cause pain, bleeding or swelling.

**Hypertrophied anal papilla** – Swollen enlarged sometimes painful or irritated anal papilla that may need to be removed if it is to troublesome.

**Impaction** – Hard stool filling the rectum and plugging the anal opening that can cause mild or severe rectal pain, constipation even diarrhea and fecal incontinence. Treated with enemas, laxatives and sometimes manual removal of the stool material. Usually prevented by adequate fiber intake.

**Infrared coagulation (IRC)** – Office treatment for internal hemorrhoids that are not too big. A focused light beam is directed on to the hemorrhoid burning a portion of it. Usually this is relatively painless.

**Internal anal sphincter** – Involuntary muscle that keeps the anal opening closed during rest, inactivity and sleep.

**Internal hemorrhoids** – Lining of the rectum that has been dragged down by bowel movements into the anal canal causing pain and bleeding.

**Intussusception** – Flopping or telescoping of the rectum due to loss of support that can block rectal emptying.

**Laparoscopy** – Surgical technique in which instruments and video cameras are placed into the abdomen through very small incisions (Band-Aid incisions). Some operations can be done inside the abdomen without making the large incision in the skin previously required.

**Large intestine (colon)** – Hollow muscular tube where waste and water from the small intestine is emptied and where the waste is stored and the water is reabsorbed into the blood stream.

**Lower GI** – Barium enema.

**Mesentery** – The tissue that attaches the intestines to the body inside the abdominal cavity. the mesentery also includes the blood vessels that carry blood to and from the intestines. The mesentery and mesenteric blood vessels must be divided to remove a portion of the intestine.

**Non-relaxing puborectalis** – Failure of the puborectalis muscle and external anal sphincter muscle to relax during attempted evacuation of the rectum which makes it difficult for the rectum to empty. Treated by pelvic muscle retraining.

**Overflow Incontinence** – Unwanted leakage of liquid or solid stool from the rectum due to hard stool impacted in the rectum. The hard stool is too big to come through the anal opening but the sphincter muscles are stretched. The colon makes mucous to try to get rid of the impaction. Liquid stool builds up above the impaction and the liquid and mucous leak out around the impaction. This is most commonly found in children and is a common cause of encopresis.

**Pancreas** – Solid organ in the upper abdomen laying on top of the backbone which produces insulin to regulate blood sugar levels and enzymes that are emptied into the intestine where they help digest food.

**Pancreatitis** – Inflammation of the pancreas causing severe pain in the abdomen and radiating to the back. It may be caused by gallstones, alcohol ingestion or it may have no apparent cause that we can find. It is treated with dietary changes, enzyme supplements and avoiding alcohol. Endoscopic ultrasound is the most sensitive medical test to identify pancreatitis. EUS can see pancreatitis even when it is missed by blood tests and CAT scans.

**Pilonidal cyst** – Cyst under the skin over the tail bone caused by hairs growing into the skin.

**Proctitis** – Inflammation of the rectum that may be due to germs or radiation therapy but in most cases we do not know the cause. It causes rectal and lower abdominal pain, urgency to move bowels, diarrhea, passage of mucous from the rectum and rectal bleeding.

**Proctoscopy** – Office diagnostic procedure in which a lighted rigid metal tube is placed into the rectum to look at the lining of the rectum.

**Pruritus ani** – Anal itching usually due to chemical irritation of the anal skin due to stool being rubbed onto it by toilet paper. Soap and vigorous washing make it worse.

**Pudendal nerve** – Nerve to the pelvic floor and anal sphincter muscles. If this nerve is damaged the sphincter muscles may be weak. Childbirth is the most common cause of damage to the pudendal nerve.

**Pudendal nerve electromyography** – Outpatient diagnostic study which measures the function of the pudendal nerve by seeing how fast it conducts and impulse along its length.

**Rectal descent** – Loss of rectal support to the pelvic bones allowing the rectum to slide down into the pelvis to such an extent that it impairs rectal emptying. Rectocele, rectal prolapse and solitary rectal ulcer are all forms of rectal descent.

**Rectal prolapse** – Loss of rectal support allowing the rectum to fall all of the way through the anal canal and protrude out of the anus.

**Rectocele** – Bulging of the rectum forward into the vagina. This bulge can fill with stool and be very hard to empty. It is caused by a loss of support of the rectum and the vagina.

**Rectopexy** – Major surgical procedure to treat rectal descent, rectal prolapse and solitary rectal ulcer in which the rectum is resuspended to the sacrum and pelvic bone.

**Rectum** – The bottom 6-8 inches of the colon.

**Rubberband ligation of internal hemorrhoids** – Office treatment of internal hemorrhoids in which a small rubber band is placed around an internal hemorrhoid. This cuts off the blood supply to the hemorrhoid and it falls of in 4-10 days. This is usually relatively painless although painful complications can sometimes occur.

**Sigmoid colon** – The 12-18 inches of colon just above the rectum. It has an "S" shape which gives it its name. It is the most common site of diverticulosis. It is located in the left lower quadrant of the belly.

**Sigmoidocele** – Bulging of the sigmoid colon into weak spots in the pelvic floor caused by inadequate support of the sigmoid colon, the rectum and the vagina. If it is causing symptoms then it can be treated by resuspending the pelvic organs from the bones of the pelvis and removing the excess sigmoid colon.

**Sigmoidoscopy** – Office diagnostic procedure that uses a fiberoptic light and camera in a flexible tube to look at the lining of the colon. The patient is awake while this is done and only the last one or two feet of the colon are examined.

**Small intestine** – Hollow muscular tube about 15-25 feet long where the nutrition of food is absorbed.

**Sphincterography** – X-ray examination of the anal muscles that measures the strength and shape of the anal sphincter.

**Sphincterotomy** – Minor surgical procedure in which some of the fibers of the internal anal sphincter are divided to take tension off of an anal fissure and allow it to heal.

**Solitary rectal ulcer** – Ulcer on the inner surface of the rectum caused by pressure pushing a floppy, redundant and inadequately supported rectal wall into the anal canal during straining to make the bowels move. It can cause pain, bleeding and the sensation that the rectum needs to be emptied. It is usually associated with difficult rectal emptying. It is not a form of colitis or Crohn's disease.

**Thrombosed external hemorrhoids** – Swollen anal skin caused by a broken blood vessel under the skin which produces a blood blister under the skin that stretches the skin causing severe pain.

**Total colectomy and ileorectal anastomosis** – Major surgical procedure in which the colon is shortened to treat severe constipation due to colonic inertia. No colostomy or bag is required.

**Transit time** – X-ray diagnostic procedure that measures how fast the intestines move food and waste through the body. This identifies people with slow colons (colonic inertia).

**Ulcerative colitis** – Inflammation of the colon with no known cause which can cause abdominal pain, diarrhea or rectal bleeding but not fistulas.

**Water hygiene** – Using water only to clean the anal area at all times. Best treatment for pruritus ani.